THE TRUTH, THE WAY
AND
THE LIFE

The Truth about Why You Are
a Slave to Sickness, the Way
to Transform Your Health, and
How to Live an Abundant Life

DR. DAVIS E. LINDSAY

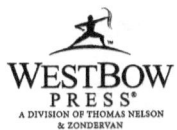

WESTBOW
PRESS®
A DIVISION OF THOMAS NELSON
& ZONDERVAN

WestBow Press books may be ordered through
booksellers or by contacting:

WestBow Press
A Division of Thomas Nelson & Zondervan
1663 Liberty Drive
Bloomington, IN 47403
www.westbowpress.com
1 (866) 928-1240

ISBN: 978-1-5127-4698-3 (sc)
ISBN: 978-1-5127-4699-0 (hc)
ISBN: 978-1-5127-4697-6 (e)

Library of Congress Control Number: 2016914320

Print information available on the last page.

WestBow Press rev. date: 1/9/2017

Contents

Acknowledgements

To my wife Kimberly, my greatest cheerleader and friend. Thank you for challenging me and questioning me, for helping me and loving me.

To my staff, patients and practice members, for supporting me, inspiring me and trusting me with your most precious asset; your health and your children's health. I am truly blessed to come into my office and help so many wonderful people.

To my colleagues in medicine, chiropractic and other health fields I appreciate your knowledge even if we don't always agree on treatment methods. Thank you for challenging me, inspiring me and supporting me.

To my parents and family for supporting me all my life and believing in me.

To God, thank you for giving me the Truth, the Way and an Abundant Life.

Introduction

My story starts as most people's stories do. My mom gave birth to me when I was quite young, and without any prompting I kept on growing. Nothing too major happened to me until I was five years old. I was learning to skate as all good Canadian kids do when I fell face first on the ice. I bit my tongue, which required stitches. I don't recommend you try that. After a couple of weeks it was fully healed, and the spiderlike black stitches that adorned my tongue had dissolved. I was back to normal, or so I thought.

Three years later I woke up one morning feeling weak and heavy with a numb and tingling left arm. This lasted for about a week before my parents took me to visit a medical doctor. He asked me to move my arm and grasp his hand, and he poked my arm to see if I could feel him touching me. I was able to do all of those things, but it just didn't feel right. He said it would probably go away on its own and not to worry about it.

Well, it didn't go away, but I just started using my right arm more and my left arm less. I had been mostly left- handed before that time, but I gradually became very right-hand dominant.

After the skating injury I started to have other problems, such as frequent nose bleeds, waking up nightly to urinate (or wetting the bed if I didn't wake up), poor eyesight, buzzing in my ear, pounding in my chest, heart arrhythmia, allergies, grinding noises in my neck, frequent sore throats, sinus infections, ringing in my ear, headaches, migraines, depression, mildly high blood pressure, frustration, fatigue, fallen arches, knee pains, and freckles (well, that's normal for redheads). These things didn't all happen at once or all the time at first.

When I was thirteen years old I went back to the medical doctor. This time he poked my arm full of holes to make me bleed and then put different kinds of drops on the punctures to see if my body reacted. We basically found out what we already knew: I was allergic to trees, grass, and pollens. The one thing we didn't know was that I had some food allergies too. The advice was to take drugs for the symptoms, but I wasn't told what caused these problems or how to correct them.

The allergy medication barely helped and always made me feel groggy. I remember finding out a few years later that the allergy drug I had been taking was discontinued due to the "side effect" of causing heart problems. That was the real eye opener for me. I didn't realize that people were the guinea pigs for drug companies. I switched to taking more natural remedies from the health food store. They had basically the same limited benefits, but I could worry less about damaging my body.

I was supposed to be in the prime of my life, and I felt horrible. In spring and summer I hated going outside, because I would be so plugged up from allergies that it was painful. It didn't seem right that I had all of these problems that my parents and brothers didn't. I figured that it couldn't have been genetic, so I struggled to find a solution to my health problems.

I decided to go to university when I was twenty years old. One morning during my freshman year I woke up in severe pain, barely able to get out of bed. It hurt to sit or stand or even lie down. I couldn't explain it. I was physically strong and fit. I was running, rowing, or weight lifting every day. After a couple of days of missed classes, I went to the campus medical clinic. The doctor looked me over for five minutes and then handed me some free drug samples and a prescription for more drugs.

By the time I was twenty, I was taking ibuprofen several

times per week, as I had a headache every day. On good days the headaches were a dull ache, and on bad days they were migraines. My ibuprofen usage eventually led to a bleeding stomach ulcer, so I stopped taking it.

I didn't want more drugs. I wanted to get healthy once and for all. I asked the doctor what the cause of the problem was and what could I do to help my body heal. He shrugged his shoulders and left the room. I was suffering and worried about my future. This university-educated man couldn't help me. No other medical doctors before him could either. I imagined my future was going to be a painful and depressing one, because I couldn't do the things I wanted to do. I had some thoughts about suicide to avoid living a life of suffering. I wanted to get better; I just didn't know how to do it.

A couple of days later would be the turning point in my life. A friend, after noticing I was suffering, suggested I go see a chiropractor. A what? I had never heard the word before and knew nothing about chiropractors. I was desperate and wanted answers, so I figured I had nothing to lose. I went to a chiropractic doctor. He told me what was wrong. He explained that the numbness and weakness and pain in my left arm were from nerve compression that probably began when I fell skating. It turns out that when I fell, my neck was jarred, causing misalignment and nerve compression. By the time our first visit was over, I already had regained some strength in my legs and had a reduction in pain. There was no miraculous instant cure or quick fix, but I had hope that I was finally on the right track. When I asked him what I could do to help myself, he gave me a handout with exercises and other advice on how to improve. It took months and many visits to recover, but it was worth it.

Before chiropractic care, I was constantly suffering. I desperately wanted to find the *truth* about health—not just a means to suppress my symptoms. I wanted a *way* to get better—not just out of pain but truly healthy. I wanted to live an *abundant life*—not just surviving day-to-day.

This book is for those who want to know the truth. The knowledge and wisdom I have compiled here have helped me and thousands of people who have sought help from me. If you learn the *truth* and follow the *way*, then you too will be able to live your *abundant life*.

Breaking Bondage

Afterward Moses and Aaron went to Pharaoh and said, "This is what the LORD, the God of Israel says: 'Let my people go...'"

—Exodus 5:1

Approximately thirty-five hundred years ago, the king of Egypt, Pharaoh, did not want to release the Israelites, who had been slaves for four hundred years. Right now many of God's people—Jews, Christians, Muslims, Buddhists, and atheists alike—are slaves to drug companies. Drug companies have convinced most people that disease is normal. They say, "Expect it. Don't try to fight it. Don't worry; we have a drug for you." They use fear to get people to inject healthy babies with toxic chemicals in vaccines, to remove body parts as a preventative measure, and to take a myriad of drugs that mask problems, create other illnesses, and keep people enslaved to more drugs. Most people believe it is normal to die between the ages of seventy-five and eighty and that it is normal for the last ten years to be miserable. This is not normal, but that is what happens when a person is a slave to false teaching.

I believe God is saying, "Enough is enough. It is time to let my people go." This book is designed to free you from slavery—the slavery of lies, deception, fear, and illness that society has been locked into for about sixty years. Most people are taking six or more medications by time they are sixty-five. Usually it starts with one medication. Then you have to take something to deal with the effects of the first one, which then leads to another and another.

I think one of the main causes of poor health today is ignorance; not having all the information necessary to make good choices. There is so much misinformation and lies about health that it is hard to know what to believe. In John 8:32 Jesus said, "...you will know the truth and the truth will set you free." The only way to be free from the slavery of illness is to know the truth.

This is how it often starts. People have some chronic pain, so they take an anti-inflammatory or a pain killer. This goes on for years until they get worse, so then they take arthritis pills or some stronger medication. Pain leads to an increase in stress hormones, so their blood pressure goes up. Then they take blood pressure medication. A chronically high level of stress hormones leads to higher cholesterol, so they also have to take some medication for that. These usually cause liver, kidney, stomach, or intestinal problems, so they take medication for that too. Then they mysteriously get cancer and are off for more drugs or surgery.

Can you see the cycle and the slavery? When will it end? It ends either when people come to their senses and realize the medication is not healing but harming them, or it ends when they die from taking the medications. Sadly, most people die much younger than they should, not realizing that they never needed the drugs in the first place and that they could have unlocked the natural healing power they already possessed.

It is easy to take prescription drugs because usually a person feels better after taking them. The fix is quick and easy, but it is a deadly snare that leads to slavery. I'm sure the Israelites didn't see the repercussions of slavery coming either, and they put up with it for a long time. After they had left and were in the desert, they longed to go back because that was what they were used to. Change can be hard at first, but it usually pays off.

Drugs don't fix any problems and they also create new problems because they are toxic in some way. Drugs don't make us healthier; they only mask symptoms. Drugs can decrease or eliminate a symptom, but the problem is still there, and after taking drugs you have one more problem than you started with, even if you feel better.

Every drug is toxic; it is a poison to the body. The body can get rid of a small amount, but just like cigarettes, drugs build up in the body and make us sick. One or two days of taking a drug is not a major problem, but once a week or once a day for weeks, months, or years will cause damage. Most people thought cigarettes were good for them sixty years ago. Heck, medical doctors and dentists even recommended them. Of course most people now know better. To be truly healthy, you must remove toxins from your body—not add them.

Three things cause all human health problems: toxicity, deficiency, and divine intervention. Except for the very small number of individuals born with genetic defects, we are programmed at birth to be healthy. For those individuals born with genetic abnormalities, the cause can also be traced back to toxicity, deficiency, or divinity. What this means is that our environment and lifestyle cause our health problems. Genetically speaking, we have not changed since humans first appeared on earth, yet our population is becoming more and more sick.

Sickness is a choice (most of the time). Many people are hurt by events or circumstances they did not choose, but maintaining one's health or deciding how to deal with illness is each person's choice. Taking drugs is a lifestyle choice. Unfortunately, many people become enslaved to drugs because of ignorance. If you don't know what healthy is, how can you ever achieve it? This has nothing to do with intelligence, but it has a lot to do with a lack of knowledge.

There is not one single health problem on this planet that is caused by a *lack* of pharmaceutical drugs! You cannot name one, because it does not exist. So why spend billions of dollars every year trying to get people healthy again with unsafe drugs that only treat *symptoms* and cause damage to vital organs? Most people in the developed parts of the world turn to drugs because most people don't know what healthy is or how to get there. When people are healthy, most of the time they don't know how to stay healthy. By the time most people hit age twenty-two, their health is already declining.

Probably the most common cause of illness today in industrialized nations is toxicity. *Toxicity* refers to either too much of something that in small amounts is not detrimental but at a certain level becomes harmful or anything that even in small doses is poisonous. Examples of toxic things include legal and illegal drugs, alcohol, tobacco, medications, pesticides, food preservatives, artificial colors, artificial flavors, MSG, bad fats, too much protein, flavor enhancers, paint fumes, plastics, aluminum cans, nonstick coatings, air pollutants, water pollutants, synthetic hormones, antibiotics, sinful behaviors, vaccinations, mercury, heavy metals, harmful thoughts, and harmful relationships. Even exercise can be toxic if a person is overtraining. If someone were to decide to run a marathon without having run even five kilometers before, running that marathon would be toxic.

The second most common cause of illness is deficiency. Examples of *deficiency* include not drinking enough water, insufficient vitamins and minerals, low fiber, not enough fruits and vegetables, not enough sunlight, not enough sleep, too little exercise, not enough healthy fats, ignoring God, loneliness, a lack of love, not enough laughter, and improper nerve function.

Divine intervention refers to times when God causes our bodies or minds to become sick or allows spiritual attacks to harm us. There are many examples in the Bible. God is the creator of all people, the earth, and the entire universe. He has the ability to make us sick or make us well. He is not some evil puppet master just wanting to mess with us. God is love. Whatever He does, He does because He loves us. He allows us to make mistakes because He gave us free will. If He were to intervene every time we made a mistake, He would be removing our free will. But there are times when He will scourge (discipline) us or remove His protection to get our attention for our own good. So if you are sick and no one can seem to figure out why, ask God. For example, breaking one of the Ten Commandments on a continual basis (bearing false witness, for example) will cause people to be spiritually sick. It may not be evident right away, but eventually it will. If you want to learn more about spiritual health, read chapter 10.

There are *three phases to health: healthy, unhealthy,* and *sick.* You are in one of those categories at any given time. Within each category is a spectrum; it's not a clear-cut jump from one phase to next. For example, a person could be just slightly unhealthy or quite unhealthy, bordering on sick. If you want to find out which category you are in, take this quiz:

- Define healthy (in one sentence without having to pause for more than four seconds to think about it).
- What are the thirteen factors you need to be healthy?
- Are you tired at the end of your workday?
- Do you nap?
- Do you get at least one cold each year?
- Are your blood pressure and resting heart rate too high?
- Do you run out of air in under thirty seconds when holding your breath?
- Are you performing stretches and exercises inconsistently or less than daily?
- Do you smoke?
- Do you drink less than two liters of water in a day?
- Do you drink pop daily?
- Is your diet low in omega-3 fatty acids?
- Do you eat less than six to seven servings of fruits and vegetables daily?
- Do you sleep less than seven or more than nine hours per night or wake up during the night?
- Are you depressed?
- Has it been more than a day since you spent time with God?
- Is there someone you need to forgive?
- Have you lost your passion for life?
- Do you replenish your healthy bacteria less than once per day?

- Is your spine abnormal? Is your nervous system malfunctioning?
- Do you have any genetic abnormalities that impair your body or mind function? (Please note that some genetic conditions are going to impair a person's health and some will not, see chapter 13 for more information)
- Are you getting less than fifteen minutes of sunshine daily?
- Do you have any pain that lasts more than three days?
- Are you taking any drugs, including prescription drugs (such as birth control), nonprescription drugs (such as daily aspirin), alcohol (more than one drink per day), or illegal drugs?
- Do you have mercury fillings or poor dental health?

If you answered "yes" or "I don't know" to any of these, then you are not healthy. If you answered no to all of these then you are probably healthy. If you want to find out how to be healthy, then keep reading.

What Is Healthy?

Healthy is when your body-mind-spirit is functioning at 100 percent. In other words, healthy is the normal function of your body-mind-spirit. We can't separate body from mind or spirit from body in this state; the three are distinct but intertwined. When all your body systems are running at 100 percent, you are healthy. Statistics show that most people are healthy up to age twenty-two, but then it's downhill from there. When a person is no longer healthy, he or she becomes either unhealthy or sick.

What Is Unhealthy?

Unhealthy is when a person's body is not functioning at normal levels, but the situation is not bad enough for the person to be outright sick. Most adults are unhealthy. The most common elements that characterize unhealthy people are stress, fatigue, stiffness, and achiness. Stress is a feeling of unease that comes in many forms, including stress to joints, stress to organs, and mental stress. When a person is toxic, deficient, or traumatized, his or her body is under stress. Spiritual stress comes when a person is not right with God. When stress hormone levels rise, blood sugars go up, blood pressure increases, platelets become stickier, breathing increases, muscle tension increases, digestion decreases, mental cognition decreases, and pupils dilate.

When a person's body is under stress and not functioning normally, fatigue sets in. Most people are so tired by the end of their workday that they don't have much energy left to cook a healthy meal, so it's store-bought microwave food or canned food or fast food. Then it's onto the couch for three hours of television, then bed, and then waking up to drag themselves to work. After work the same cycle is repeated day in and day out. That's not living; that's merely existing. Too much stress for too long leads to the third phase of health, which is sickness.

What Is Sick?

It's easy to know when you are *sick*; you don't have to guess. Sick, however, doesn't just mean you have a head cold or are throwing up. Sick is when you have a noticeable symptom or illness. If you have diabetes, cancer, high blood pressure, migraine headaches, back pain, allergies, and so on, you know you are sick.

Most people can remember a day when they were healthy: the energy that didn't seem to quit, the ease of movement, mental clarity and pure happiness, and being able to use their bodies to do whatever they chose. That's where the frustration sets in. Remembering the "good old days" leads to frustration: "I remember when I had tons of energy and felt great." Sound familiar? If you find yourself saying, "I think I'm healthy" or "I'm healthy except for …" then you are unhealthy. You don't guess when you are healthy. If you truly know what health is, then you know when you have it. Most unhealthy people are afraid of getting sick because they don't know how to prevent it. They tend to "knock on wood" if they have not been sick for a while. I guess they think good health has to do with good luck. Unhealthy people give up things they like to do because they feel worse if they do it. "As long as I don't go bowling, I'm fine," or "I'm healthy now that I don't run anymore" are all signs of unhealthiness.

Why is it that someone can be aging gracefully at one hundred, but somewhere else a teenager is stricken with cancer and dies? We may never be able to fully answer that question, but the more you know about health, the better your odds of living to one hundred or older.

Research shows that we can change our health if we give our bodies the right tools. Diseases, such as cancer, heart disease, osteoporosis, arthritis, allergies, asthma, and diabetes, can be reversed! We have to remove the toxicity, eliminate the deficiencies, deal with any trauma, and get right with God. Then and only then will a person truly be healthy.

I know that this may sound too simple or too good to be true, but the reality is our bodies want to bring us back to homeostasis, balance, and health. If we are too hot, we sweat; if we are too cold, we shiver. God designed our bodies to heal themselves. Our bodies are inherently intelligent; we need to allow them to do what they were designed to do—not stop the symptoms with some chemical or drug.

According to government statistics, 83 percent of people aged sixty-five to seventy-nine are taking some kind of prescription medication on a regular basis.[1] If you factor in over-the-counter medication, it is almost 100 percent. Healthy people don't need drugs! We have more technology, more knowledge, and more money than ever, but as a population we are sicker. It's time to face the numbers; the statistics don't lie. We can keep throwing more money at the drug companies and hope that will help, or we can accept the fact that we need to change.

I'm not saying we need to do away with the medical system, but it obviously needs to change. Severe trauma and emergencies are where the medical approach is best utilized. Medical doctors save lives every day. My own wife would be dead right now if it weren't for medical physicians and drugs, so I'm grateful for that. The drugs help to treat severe sickness. After the crisis is over, the person goes from being sick to unhealthy. That is when most people assume they are healthy. It feels a lot better to go from sick to unhealthy, so it is easy to conclude that this improved state means the person is healthy. Again, drugs *cannot* get you healthy. Remember the definition of healthy is when your body-mind-spirit is functioning at 100 percent. That means no drugs. Every drug is a toxin that affects the body in negative ways if taken long enough.

Drugs don't actually fix the problem; they mask the symptoms. Now you have two problems, the original one you are taking drugs for and now the added stress to your body of this toxic drug. There are no safe drugs. Avoid them as much as you can.

Most people today follow the *allopathic model of health*. It's also called "modern medicine." In the allopathic model, the body is seen as a genetic time bomb that is designed to breakdown and is inherently weak and in need of human intervention to make it work right. Since it is preprogrammed to fail, there is no correcting the cause of poor health in the allopathic model; drugs are then offered to help alleviate a person's suffering. When an organ is failing, it is either removed or, if possible, replaced. When a person no longer has symptoms, he or she is considered to be "healthy." When symptoms return, that person returns to a medical physician for more drugs. Diseases are treated rather than people. Allopathic medicine sees aging as a disease that brings with it all kinds of sickness and suffering. It's not a very rosy outlook is it? This model works very well in dealing with acute health emergencies, such as severe bleeding, stroke, heart attack, fractured bones, and poisoning. In other words, this is emergency-room care. This model is not appropriate for health maintenance, optimal wellness or prevention of degenerative illness or diseases.

Think of medicine like the fire department, only call them when your house is on fire. You wouldn't want your house being hosed down with water every day other wise it will suffer water damage, rot or mould. The fire department is not going to improve the health of your house, we need carpenters and other tradespeople for that.

On the other hand, the *wellness model of health* is based on the fact that the human body is programmed for health. Genetically our bodies want to keep us healthy. The role of the doctor in this model is to remove any interference preventing the body from healing itself, correct any deficiencies, and remove any toxicity that is causing illness. The person with the symptoms is treated as a whole rather than treating the symptoms a person has. Symptoms are seen as the body's response to illness instead of viewing the symptoms as the problem. The body is governed by an Innate Intelligence (the nervous system) that controls and coordinates all structures and functions within the body-mind-spirit. In this model, good health is expected throughout all stages of life. This model works very well for chronic degenerative illness and prevention of illness. This model may not be appropriate for severe or acute emergencies.

Allopathic Model	Wellness Model
Sickness care	Wellness care
Treat symptoms	Address root causes
Reductionist	Holistic
Suppressive	Vitalistic
Dogmatic	"Pain free does not equal healthy"

Allopathic Model	Wellness Model
"No pain, no problem"	Unlimited Potential
Limited Potential	Moving toward healthy
Moving away from illness	Care for chronic illness and
Emergency treatment	degenerative disease

You will discover as you read this book that healing comes from God and within yourself. We are designed to be healthy. Our body-mind-spirit will always do what's best for us. In other words, the symptoms are not bad; they are actually our body-mind-spirit dealing with the illness.

Instead of asking doctors to fix you, you need to be asking, *"What do I need to do to allow my body to heal? What am I deficient in, how can I eliminate toxins, and how can I get right with God?"* Your body is not like a car you can drop off at the mechanic and pick up when it's fixed. Healing is a process, and *you* have the greatest impact on *your* health. Only you and God can heal you. The word *doctor* means teacher, not healer. I've helped many patients' lives improve, but I haven't healed a single one.

Just because you are pain free doesn't mean you are healthy. The day before a heart attack, a person's heart feels fine, but research shows that in most heart attacks the problem has been present for years. Finally the body can no longer compensate, and the heart severely malfunctions. If a person knew a heart attack was coming, he or she would check in to the hospital the day before it happened. So don't make the fatal mistake millions of people do every year and assume, "If I don't hurt, I don't have a problem." This erroneous belief probably will lead to your early death.

God says in Genesis 6:3, "My Spirit will not contend with man forever, for he is mortal; his days will be 120 years." Science agrees that approximately 120 years appears to be the upper limit of human life. So why are so many people dying by age seventy-five or eighty? It's not bad luck or bad genes. It is education and lifestyle. What we don't know can kill us. We don't know what God has in store for us, but if we take care of our health, we should live well into our nineties, one hundreds, and beyond.

Good health or sickness is based on choices. We are a product of all our choices. We choose to be healthy by making healthy choices. We choose to be sick by making sick (bad) choices. I have chosen not to smoke. That is a healthy choice. I choose to limit my sugars, another healthy choice. This does not make me a better person, just healthier. In each chapter you will see that you are given the choice of healthy versus sick. There are no other options. If you are healthy and start making sick choices, you will become unhealthy and then, eventually, you will become sick. On the contrary, if you are sick and start making healthy choices, you will become unhealthy and then, eventually, healthy. Sometimes people make too many sick choices for too long and can never be healthy again, but as long as you are alive and desire to change, you probably can. Even if you only improve your health by 5 percent, that's still better than getting 5 percent worse. So think positively, and don't expect to change overnight. Most people don't get sick overnight; it takes years of bad choices to get there.

Wherever possible, I take the Bible as the absolute truth on any subject because no one has ever been able to disprove any of it. When I am unable to find the answer in the Bible, I use what science says if it matches with the character and Spirit of God.

If you don't believe in an all-knowing, all-present, loving God, don't worry; you will still gain insight as to how you can improve your health. My goal is to give you Truth so that you can be set free, to show you the Way to live healthy, and to give you the opportunity to have the Abundant Life you deserve; the rest is up to you.

2

Sunlight

> For God made two great lights, the sun and the moon, to shine down upon the earth ... God set these lights in the heavens to light the earth, to govern the day and the night and to separate the light from the darkness. And God saw that it was good.
>
> —Genesis 1:16–18 NIV

We need the sun. God put it there for a reason. If the sun were bad, He would have told us to hide from it. God said, " ...it was good." We have been living in a society that has been told to fear the sun. The sun causes cancer, or so we've been led to believe. It is not true. Who do you believe—God (the creator of the sun) or people (His creation)?

Don't forget the sunscreen, right? Wrong!

Most sunscreen lotions are filled with toxic chemicals that block UVA and UVB rays. We need sun. Sunlight is the primary means of producing vitamin D_3 in our bodies, which converts vitamin D_3 into vitamin D. It is true that too much sunlight can cause burns, but if we use good sense we can avoid that. We need around thirty minutes of sun exposure daily. Dark-skinned people will need thirty to sixty minutes per day, and fair-skinned people will need fifteen to thirty minutes. After that it's a good idea to cover up, but not with lotions. It's also best to be careful when the UV rays of the sun are at their peak strength, which varies slightly depending on where you live from eleven o'clock in the morning to four o'clock in the afternoon.

We need vitamin D for several reasons. Vitamin D is needed for our bodies to absorb calcium. When a person has normal vitamin D levels, he or she doesn't need to consume as much calcium, because calcium absorption is more efficient. Vitamin D is added to milk for that very reason; however, fortified milk is a poor source of vitamin D and calcium, as I will discuss in more detail in chapter 3.

Calcium is vital for bones, teeth, muscle, and nerve-cell function. When a person is not getting enough calcium, the brain will release hormones to increase the breakdown of bone to increase the level of calcium in the blood. In essence, calcium is robbed from the bones to keep the other vital functions going. If this occurs for too long, severe bone and muscular disorders, including osteoporosis, develop.[2] When the body is deficient in nutrients it will take them from somewhere less vital to maintain homeostasis.

Our bodies will maintain our health in other ways too. For example, if a person is cold, the brain triggers the hairs on the arms and legs to contract to increase heat production and trap a layer of warmer air around the body. If that doesn't work, the muscles are told to shiver, causing friction and heat. Then the brain decreases the flow of blood to the extremities in an effort to preserve core temperature. If a person continues to get colder, almost all blood is kept in the trunk to keep the vital organs alive. This leads to hypothermia, which is a form of shock. The brain is willing to sacrifice the arms and legs so that the person might live.

Vitamin D is important in mental function as well. During the winter months, the sun's rays are not strong enough to stimulate vitamin D in the skin. In North America, north of the thirty-fifth parallel, which is anywhere north of Sacramento, California, and Washington, DC, the sun's rays are not strong enough from October to April to stimulate vitamin D production. This includes all of Canada and the northern European countries, such as the United Kingdom, Sweden, Norway, and northern Russia, to name a few.

Not getting enough sunlight can cause depression. If the depression occurs mainly in the winter months, it is termed SAD or seasonal affective disorder. This is probably due to low serotonin levels and inadequate levels of vitamin D in the diet, which manifests itself as depression in the winter when the individual is no longer receiving vitamin D from the sun. Research using full spectrum and bright lights in the home throughout the day, but especially during the morning, shows a *decrease* in major depression by up to 57 percent.[3] The optimal time to get bright light is before eight o'clock in the morning. A person needs to aim for five thousand lux hours per day. If you had a five-thousand-lux light you would need to use it for an hour, or you could use a ten-thousand-lux light for thirty minutes.[4] Both methods would give you the same dosage of light.

A lack of sunlight also leads to an increase in carbohydrate cravings—seemingly a sign of the body's effort to bring up its energy levels. Unfortunately, this leads to weight gain, because people don't usually go for healthy carbohydrates, such as an apple or a carrot; they usually eat crackers, bread, or muffins.

Why doesn't everyone in northern areas suffer from depression in the winter? Don't forget: there are twelve other keys to unlocking health. When sunlight levels are lower, make sure to maintain an active lifestyle, which will also help to keep serotonin levels regulated. Getting cold-water fish oil in the winter can keep your vitamin D levels normal and give your brain the essential fatty acids that it needs.

People in northern regions also have higher rates of multiple sclerosis (MS), which is probably due to decreased sunlight.[5] The exception to this is people in Norway. In other parts of the world, the farther north a population is, the higher the rate of MS. Researchers have found that Norwegians who take cod liver oil or eat fish three or more times per week have lower rates of MS even when they spend less time outdoors. They also found that children who increased their outdoor activity level during summer months had lower rates of MS.[6]

It is not a coincidence that in areas where sunlight is less intense, God provided fish to give us the vitamin D we need. Cold-water fish have high levels of vitamin D, and cold-water fish are found in places with lower levels of sun. According to the National Institutes of Health, one tablespoon of cod liver oil will supply more than enough vitamin D for the day.[7] Salmon, tuna, sardines, and mackerel are also good sources of vitamin D. Conversely, tropical fish don't have the same high levels of vitamin D, but since they are found in places with higher sunlight levels, it's not necessary for people living in these places to supplement with fish oil. It also seems that a person can get more vitamin D than needed in the summer and store it in the liver for winter. As the winter months drag on, the vitamin D bank becomes depleted. When spring arrives the cycle can start all over again. This is partially why many people feel better in the spring: they have more energy, they feel more alert, and they feel more alive.

The incidence of melanoma (skin cancer) has increased over the last one hundred years, which directly coincides with a larger percentage of the population working indoors. Only around 10 percent of the population in North America works outdoors, whereas one hundred years ago it was closer to 75 percent. It is interesting to note that while the percentage of the population spending less time in the sun has increased, more people are suffering from skin cancers. More and more studies are showing that sunscreen use does not decrease cancer rates; in fact the rates of melanoma go up with sunscreen use.[8] Other research shows that skin cancers decrease in people who perform regular exercise (more about that in chapter 4).

Natural Skin Protection

There are ways to protect yourself from the sun without using toxic chemicals. The safest method is to get indoors or into the shade. Long loose clothing and umbrellas work great also. One spring I was in Atlanta, Georgia, and I saw many local dark-skinned people using umbrellas, not because of rain but because of sun. That is much smarter than applying the damaging chemicals in sunscreen lotions. A client who was born and raised in the Philippines sixty years ago mentioned that as a child she would avoid the intense part of the day (ten o'clock in the morning to about half-past three in the afternoon) and wear longer clothing and large hats to protect herself. Most people she knew practiced this common-sense behavior.

There are several companies that manufacture clothing offering higher UPF (ultraviolet protection factor) ratings. Sunsolutions.com, platypusaustralia.com, and sunprotective-clothing.com from Canada have been selling hats, shirts, jackets, and pants for years that can allow you to be in the sun up to fifty times longer than if you were uncovered.

Safe Lotions

Most sunscreens contain toxins; however, there are some companies that use fewer than others. A good practice is to seek out antioxidants, such as vitamin E, vitamin C, and beta-carotene, which protect the skin against overexposure without any harmful side effects. These can be used either orally or topically. If you would like a safer sunscreen because you just can't avoid being in the sun, then go to your local health food store. They usually have a variety of less toxic sunscreens. Instead of using harmful chemicals, such as octysalicylate and homosalate, they use titanium dioxide (a mineral that deflects the sun's rays from the skin) or a mixture of green tea, shea butter, and white camella oil. The Environmental Working Group has an excellent website that lists hundreds of sunscreens and the toxins they contain (www.ewg.org). The best and safest natural skin lotion is coconut butter or coconut oil. This same client I mentioned earlier also mentioned that the people of the Philippines and other hot places use coconut oil as a safe and healthy skin lotion. God provides us with everything we need.

Sometimes the toxins sound safe. Recently, a scientific panel from the National Institutes for Health found that vitamin A (retinyl palmitate), which is found in forty percent of sunscreens, speeds the development of skin tumors when applied to skin in the presence of sunlight.[9] That's why I don't use any sunscreen lotions.

It's not the sun that causes skin cancer. It could be a combination of toxic lifestyle choices, such as sunscreens, cosmetics, overuse of tanning beds, low water intake, poor diet, inadequate exercise, not enough sun, and poor nerve function.[10]

Whether skin is burned because of too much heat (fire) or too much sun, our bodies have the ability to heal themselves. In order for proper healing to occur, the right nutrients must be present (healthy eating), the body must have good blood flow (from exercise), and the body must have normal nerve function (cell replacement).

Skin health comes from the inside out. Skin cells are nourished by the blood supply coming from within the body. The skin's outer surface is already *dead*, so why are so many people trying to get healthier skin by wearing expensive lotions? I'm sure we've all seen the dog food commercials touting how the use of their dog food will give your dog a nice shiny coat. It's what is in the food that causes the fur on the dog to shine—not some special shampoo. The same is true for us as well: if you want to look good on the outside, be careful of what you put inside.

We need the sun. God put the sun in the sky for us. Plants wither and die if they don't get enough sun, and so do people. Plants will burn if they get too much sun, and so will people. Get enough sunlight, and get out of the sun when you have had enough; don't cover your body in toxic chemicals so you can stay out longer. The more you are exposed to the sun, the longer you will be able to stay in the sun. After six o'clock in the evening and before nine o'clock in the morning you can get hours of sun without burning; the middle of the day is when you have to be careful.

Sunlight stimulates the production of melanin in the skin. That is why a person will tan or get darker skin after sun exposure. Tanning is not a bad thing. Sun exposure is like exercise for your skin. If you get too much all at once, you will be sore. If you gradually work up your sun exposure, you will be fine. Dark-skinned people can withstand more sun and need more sunlight to get their daily intake.

The reason why the people who live in sunny areas have dark skin is to allow them to be in the sun for longer periods of time. Light-skinned people come from less sunny places, such as northern Europe. This makes sense; light-skinned people can get their vitamin D levels replaced with less sun exposure. God does not make any mistakes; He knows what he is doing. It's not good for dark-skinned people to live in areas that are not sunny, because they are designed to be in the sun longer. If you have dark skin and are living in a northern area, get outside as much as possible and make sure you get your vitamin D in the winter.

The Inuit of the Arctic Circle and the Sami of Lapland, both of whom have darker skin, are exceptions to this rule. According to researchers, because they retain a high vitamin D diet from eating mostly cold-water fish and other seafood, their bodies didn't need to adapt to the decreased daylight. Instead of becoming pale like the Europeans, to absorb more UV for vitamin D they retained their darker skin. The grain-based diet of northern Europeans is deficient in vitamin D, so light-skinned people require more vitamin D from the sun. It turns out that wheat also contains a protein that decreases vitamin D synthesis in the skin, thereby increasing the need for vitamin D either from the sun or from other foods.[11]

Just like other animals on this planet, we all have optimal environments. For some fish it's fresh water, and for others it's salt water. It is better for people to live in their optimal environment. If you love the sun and feel depressed when it's gone, move to a sunnier climate as so many birds and other people do each winter. Given wheat's impairment to vitamin D synthesis and Westerners' general avoidance of the sun, most Westerners are vitamin D deficient. Given this fact, minimize wheat consumption and get a safe amount of sun exposure, and you will see your energy, mental health, and physical health improve.

Other Benefits of the Sun

The sun also emits infrared and x-rays. Infrared saunas are very popular for detoxification and weight loss. Sweating is a natural and necessary activity, but you are better off exercising to create sweat rather than sitting in a sauna, unless you have a limitation. Again, if you live in a cold climate during the winter, an infrared sauna can be great way to sweat out toxins.

Far infrared rays also have the ability to improve our immune systems and kill cancer cells. According to cancer specialist Dr. Nobuhiro Yoshimizu, far infrared rays help our bodies get rid of cancer cells. He recommends a sauna for forty to sixty minutes three times per day at 70 degrees Celsius to treat cancer. If our bodies get too cold (just 1 degree below normal), enzymes and immune function decrease.

It used to be thought that any amount of x-ray or ionizing radiation was harmful—the less x-ray, the better. Well, research has shown that this assumption is not true. It appears that some radiation is actually beneficial in destroying damaged cells and cancer cells in our bodies. Dr. Yoshimizu also uses low level x-rays to treat cancer. Apparently people who live at higher elevations (the Rockies) have a 15 to 25 percent lower cancer death rate than people at lower elevations.

The higher elevation subjects people to higher levels of radiation.[12] Other studies have shown that low-level x-rays are beneficial. There is a point where more x-ray is neither good nor harmful, but beyond that level, the radiation starts to be harmful.[13]

Sunglasses

Most people think they need sunglasses to protect their eyes from the sun. Did Moses wear sunglasses? No. And he lived to be 120 years old with good eyesight. Deuteronomy 34:7 says, "Moses was one hundred and twenty years old when he died, yet his eyes were not weak nor his strength gone."

Moses and the Israelites wandered around the desert for forty years without sunglasses. They most definitely had head coverings to shade their eyes. That's the best way to keep bright sun out of your eyes without altering the wavelength of light shining on your eyes.

Sunglasses could actually be causing cataracts by denying the skin of the eyes (corneas) from receiving the full light as God designed it. Just as our skin needs sunlight for vitamin D, so do our eyes. The less you wear sunglasses, the better.

There are times when shielding the eyes might be beneficial or necessary. For example, if you fly airplanes or are on the water, I would recommend that you protect your eyes.

If you are going to wear sunglasses, buy good-quality ones. Cheap glasses can cause more harm, because they don't actually filter the sun; they just shade the eyes, causing the pupils to open more to let more sunlight in. Normally, in bright light our pupils get smaller to decrease the amount of light coming in, but with sunglasses on, the pupils stay large.

To summarize, too little sun is detrimental, a moderate amount of sun is necessary and beneficial, and too much sun is harmful.

God put the sun in the sky. We need the sun in order to be healthy. With some common sense guidelines, the sun can be enjoyed and not feared. If we get the right amount, along with having the other keys to optimal health, we can thrive.

Our eyes are mostly made of water, so we need to stay hydrated. In the next chapter you will learn how much and what kind of water you need for optimal health.

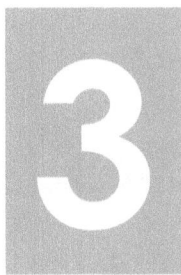

Water

Jesus answered, "Everyone who drinks this water will be thirsty again, but whoever drinks the water I give him will *never* thirst. Indeed, the water I give him will become in him a spring of water welling up to eternal life."
—John 4:13–14 NIV, emphasis mine

The Truth about Bottled Water and Why You Shouldn't Buy It

It goes without saying that we need water. After all, we are approximately two-thirds water. Adequate water is needed for gas exchange in the lungs as well as food digestion, absorption, and elimination. Water is necessary for elimination of toxins through feces, urine, and sweat. Water is needed for cellular growth, repair, and regeneration. Water is needed for the function and repair of all avascular tissues, including tendons, ligaments, cartilage, joints, and spinal discs. Our brains are roughly 85 percent water!

If you are reading this book and still aren't convinced that God exists, just stop and think about the brain for a moment. The brain is 85 percent water yet controls every cell in the body simultaneously! We are talking hundreds of trillions of cells all being coordinated by something that is almost completely water, the rest of which is mainly fat. The average blueberry is also 85 percent water, but I don't know any blueberries that can talk, walk, remember, play piano, sleep, love, or write poetry.[14]

The cerebrospinal fluid that surrounds the brain and spinal cord is almost completely made of water also. Water is necessary for life.

What is the best kind of water, and how much do we need daily? We need water that contains minerals. If you look at most bottled water, it will say demineralized or remineralized. The *dirty little secret* that the bottled water industry doesn't want you to know is that they are using reverse osmosis to purify tap water. That's right: you are buying tap water in a bottle that has all the essential minerals removed. That's what they mean by demineralized. The reason it tastes and smells better is that they have removed the chlorine. A simple charcoal filter will do that for a fraction of the cost without removing the minerals.

Remineralized water has gone through the same process, except they will add back a small portion of the minerals. Usually about four or five minerals are added back. This is only slightly better than demineralized water. Natural spring water contains forty or more minerals, depending on the source.[15]

When the minerals are removed, the water becomes acidic. This is fine for washing clothes or dishes but not for drinking. You can purchase a simple home testing kit (litmus paper) to determine the acidity of your water.

We used to purchase demineralized bottled water from a local bottling company. The bottled water we drank was city tap water that was run through filtration and reverse osmosis to remove all toxins, including fluoride and chlorine. The bottled water smelled and tasted better, but it lacked minerals. We purchased a whole home dechlorination machine and an under-the-counter reverse osmosis water filter for drinking water. It cost more initially, but within a year we were saving money on bottled water. Plus, we no longer had to deal with those pesky bottles.

This still didn't solve the problem of demineralization. If you are drinking two liters of water per day, you will need to get roughly one teaspoon of sea salt or crystal salt every day. Do *not* use regular salt; it is unhealthy (more on this later).

The healthiest water is clean spring water or well water from a clean underground spring. If you have your own well or get water from a creek, make sure to test it for contaminants.

Why Cows Are Smarter Than People

Have you ever wondered why cattle don't drink milk? Only the young calves drink cow's milk, so where does the mother cow get the calcium from so that she can pass it on to her young through her milk? She gets it from her food (grass) and water. Not only does the cow's diet supply her with enough calcium to keep her large bones strong, but she also has enough to give to her young. Don't believe the lies that you need milk to get enough calcium for strong bones. There certainly is a significant amount of calcium in dairy products, but you don't have to consume dairy products to get enough calcium if you are drinking healthy water and eating the proper foods, which will be discussed in the next chapter. According to Health Canada, we can get up to 30 percent of our daily calcium needs from drinking one and a half liters of water per day.[16]

How Much Water Should You Drink Each Day?

So now you know that you need mineral water. You can buy natural mineral water instead of demineralized water, but how much water should you drink each day?

Well, that depends on the weather, your body size, and your activity level. If you were to drink roughly eight glasses or two liters of water per day, you would probably be getting enough. If you are very active or sweating a lot during the day, increase your water intake. Drink cool (not cold) water on hot days. If you drink alcohol or caffeine or are taking diuretics (substances that cause you to lose water), you will need to drink more water.

The first thing you should put into your body every day is a glass of water. If you are going to exercise, have some fresh fruit juice also. Most people are unhealthy and feel tired when they wake up, so the first thing they do is drink coffee to "get going." Did you know being low on water (dehydrated) can make you feel tired and hungry?

Watch out for overheating in the summer months. When the humidity is high, temperatures in the high eighties (over twenty-seven degrees Celsius) can be dangerous, and when the humidity is low, temperatures in the high nineties (over thirty-two degrees Celsius) can be dangerous.

Here are some early warning signs of heat-related illness:

- Feeling dizzy or faint
- Going to the bathroom less often than usual
- Producing darker and/or yellower urine
- Experiencing labored breathing, sometimes accompanied by a pounding heart
- Suffering from a headache and/or painful muscle spasms
- Experiencing nausea and/or excessive sweating

If you exercise in the heat, make sure you drink somewhere between half a litre and one litre (one quart) of cool fluids each hour. You can make your own inexpensive and healthy sports drink by mixing five hundred milliliters(2 cups) of orange juice with five hundred milliliters of water and two or three pinches of sea salt. If you are exercising for under one hour, just water will do. If you are exercising beyond an hour or if you work outside all day, make sure you are getting a little bit of salt (provided that you don't use a lot of salt in your food already).

If people drink only demineralized water without adding necessary minerals to their diets, they can become quite ill. During a consultation, an individual told me she had been in the emergency room the previous week because she had

26

been so weak, lethargic, and off balance that she could hardly walk or talk. Her blood tests showed that her mineral levels were severely low. After some IV minerals, she was doing much better; however, she still had some loss of feeling in her hands and feet (peripheral neuropathy). She didn't know why this happened, so I asked her how much water she was drinking. Her reply was five cups per day. Then I asked her what kind of water, and she told me that it was bottled water (reverse osmosis). That was the problem: she wasn't getting any minerals, so gradually her body became depleted and her nervous system almost shut down. If we don't get enough minerals, our hearts can stop also: we need minerals for muscle contractions.

Determining Your Water Needs

How many elephants have been told how much water to drink? Answer: none. Have you ever had to tell your cat or dog how much to drink? Of course not; animals listen to their bodies and drink when they need to. However, most people don't drink enough water because they are drinking other liquids instead. Many people are so out of tune with their bodies that they don't know when they are thirsty. In time, you can regain the ability to understand when you need more water. If you are thirsty, drink water or herbal tea. Organic coffee without any added sugar or cream is also fine; just keep it to one cup every four days or less so that you don't become addicted to caffeine, which is a brain stimulant. Also, don't drink coffee after dinner or you won't be able to rest properly.

As for specialty waters, I need to warn you to avoid them. These waters have flavors and vitamins and other things added to them (in other words, toxins). They are *not* healthy.

To find out how much water you need after exercise, have a glass of water when you first get up in the morning and then weigh yourself. After exercising for one hour, weigh yourself again to see how much weight you have lost by sweating.

One kilogram of water equals one liter. So if you are one kilogram lighter (two pounds), you have lost one liter (thirty-two fluid ounces) of water. Of course you can't have eaten from the time you weigh yourself until after the exercise. Remember that you should add a slight amount of salt after exercise or during if you exercise for ninety minutes or more at a time or if it is hot or humid. It's also best to slightly overestimate how much water you are going to need. So, for example, if you have lost one kilogram during exercise, drink 1.2 litres of water or 20 percent more than you lost.[17]

Most people will actually be shorter by bedtime because they will have lost a small amount of water from between the discs in their spines, which offers another way to see if you are dehydrated. Check your height in the morning and then again by bedtime. Dehydration is not the only reason a person might become shorter: abnormal posture, bulging discs, muscle tension, or vertebral subluxations (misalignment) can also lead to a loss of height (more about this in chapter 11).

The Body Has a Water-Rationing System

When a person is low on water, the body compensates by "borrowing" water from certain areas. In an effort to keep blood volume up, water is taken out of the discs in the spine. If water level decreases to the point where blood volume decreases, the blood becomes thicker, which puts higher stress on the heart. In other words, water is a blood thinner. Why take a drug to thin the blood when you can safely drink more water. Rationing is activated when a person does not drink enough water. The first places water delivery is eliminated are to the spinal discs, ligaments, joints, and cartilages. Second to lose its water supply when dehydrated is the digestive system, and last are the brain and nervous system. Too little water, and the person dies.

Another way to recognize dehydration or lack of water is to look at your lips. If you have dry, cracked, or chapped lips, you are likely dehydrated. If your lips are dry, drink more water. I will also discuss in chapter 8 how to find a healthy lip balm.

The Pettibon Biomechanics Institute has joined other researchers in finding that fluids can be pumped in and out of the spinal discs. This allows for the elimination of waste products, the drawing in of nutrients, pain reduction, spinal correction, and improved spinal function.

The spinal discs are mainly water, so they are a good source for the body to draw from. Unfortunately, losing one millimeter of disc height from each spinal disc causes a person to lose twenty-three millimeters (nearly one inch) in height! In the short term, this solves a problem of having a low volume of blood plasma, but unfortunately the loss of disc height can lead to spinal problems. Now if a person's spine is normal, losing one millimeter from each disc, especially in the lower back, isn't going to pose a major problem. However, if the discs are already abnormally squished due to a disc injury or improper positioning of the spine (subluxations), then losing one millimeter in disc height can lead to headaches, pain anywhere along the spine, or radiating pain, numbness, or tingling along the nerves to the hands or feet. If you find you get headaches when you are dehydrated, have your spine evaluated by a chiropractor (with x-rays) to see if there is abnormal disc compression.

When you start to drink more water, you might also need to increase salt intake. If the big muscles, especially in the legs, cramp at night, this could be due to inadequate sea salt consumption. Slowly increase sea salt intake over several days until the cramping is eliminated. If you ingest too much salt, your feet will start to swell, and salt cravings will disappear. Reduce sea salt intake until the feet aren't swelling and there is no leg cramping. (Reminder: Consult a licensed health care provider for your own specific concerns. This is general advice only.)

There are other important minerals needed for proper electrolyte balance. Calcium, magnesium, and potassium are the most studied. We need calcium in conjunction with vitamin D, which isn't a problem during the summer, but make sure you get supplemental vitamin D in the winter, as discussed in the last chapter. Magnesium protects the lining of arteries, helps build bone mass, and prevents the calcification of soft tissues. It is also involved in energy-production pathways. If a person is deficient in magnesium, nerve and muscle impulses will be weak, leading to irritability, nervousness, depression, dizziness, muscle weakness, twitching, and premenstrual syndrome (PMS). It's best not to take calcium and magnesium together, as they compete for binding sites. In other words, they fight to get into the bloodstream at the same time, and there can only be one winner. Potassium is necessary for a healthy nervous system and regular heart rhythm. It helps prevent strokes, maintains proper water balance, decreases blood pressure, and promotes proper muscle function.[18]

As I mentioned earlier, use only sea salt; almost all the essential minerals have been stripped away from regular table salt. Sea salt is salt in its natural state, which has many minerals. Sea salt has iodine in it, so you don't have to worry about your thyroid being deficient. A good sea salt will have more than fifty minerals in it.

When most people think about salt, they have a negative association. Table salt is basically sodium, chloride, and iodine and is not healthy in that state. Too much salt has been shown to increase blood pressure and deplete calcium. Sea salt doesn't have the same negative effects as table salt, however. Think of table salt as the white bread of salt. White flour has had almost all the nutrients stripped away and is *not* healthy. Whole grain flours still retain many of the nutrients and are beneficial. In the same way, whole sea salt is healthy, but that doesn't mean it should be overused.

Jesus said, "*Salt is good*, but if it loses its saltiness, how can you make it salty again? *Have salt in yourselves* and be at peace with each other" (Mark 9:50, emphasis mine). Two thousand years ago, people didn't go through the trouble to strip away minerals from salt. Jesus was talking about sea salt, and He said it "is good." Sea salt enhances the flavor of food and is not a strong, harsh tasting salt. Those people listening to Him at that time knew that salt was an enhancer and a natural, safe preservative. Jesus wanted His followers to be a positive influence on their communities and to enhance and preserve the lives of those around them. I also believe Jesus was giving us some health advice along with some spiritual truth.

Water Acidity

Another important factor to consider when drinking water is the pH or acidity of the water. On the pH scale, the lower the number, the more acidic something is, and the higher the number (up to fourteen), the more alkaline it is. A pH of 7 is considered neutral. Our blood pH level should be 7.4. Drinking acidic water causes our bodies to take minerals from our tissues to try to counteract the acidity. If this goes on for too long, a person can become osteoporotic. This means that your bones don't get the calcium they need, so they become thinner in order for your body to neutralize the acid. If our bodies didn't do this, we would die from the acidity of our blood.

You can easily test your drinking water, saliva and urine by purchasing pH strips from a health food store or online. If your water is acidic, remove the chlorine with a charcoal filter or add lemon/lime juice to the water. Although citrus fruits contain citric acid, they are alkaline—as are all other fruits and vegetables. Another option is to purchase a water ionizer, which can change the pH of your water. Don't make your water too alkaline either. Your water should have a pH level between seven and eight.

A good rule of thumb to always remember is that God doesn't make mistakes, and people will *never* improve on God's creation.

Fluoride

For five decades now we've been told that we need fluoride to protect our teeth from cavities, but what we haven't been told is that fluoride is toxic. Fluoride in high enough concentrations (four parts per million) causes *dental fluorosis*, a condition that leaves the teeth blackened, pitted, and weak. Fluoride also causes damage to the skeleton, a painful and sometimes crippling condition called *skeletal fluorosis*. According to the Centers for Disease Control in 2005, 32 percent of children in the US had dental fluorosis from overexposure to fluoride.

The worst part of all of this is that there are no good studies showing any significant benefit from drinking water with fluoride in terms of preventing tooth decay. And we especially don't need it added to our water supply. Many communities pay to add fluoride to their city water. Then people pay for fluoride toothpaste, and then they go to a dentist for topical fluoride. The only one of those ideas that makes any sense at all is putting fluoride directly on the teeth. If you want fluoride, don't drink it. According to the CDC, some research shows that putting fluoride directly on the teeth can strengthen enamel, but why expose yourself to toxins?

Studies have been done comparing communities that add fluoride and ones that don't, and often the cities that do *not* add fluoride have fewer cavities. According to the World Health Organization, western European countries have the same rate of dental cavities as areas that add fluoride to their water; importantly, 97 percent of western European countries do *not* add fluoride. Adding fluoride to tap water is basically drugging people without their consent. It should be illegal.

My children have not used fluoride toothpaste, and I haven't used it for many years now, and we don't have any new cavities. We also filter our water to get the fluoride and chlorine out, and we don't get the fluoride treatment on our teeth when we go to the dentist either.

If fluoride can damage the skeleton and teeth, imagine

what it can do to the rest of you. As Dr. John Colquhoun has said, "Common sense should tell us that if a poison circulating in a child's body can damage the tooth-forming cells, then other harm is also likely."[19] The fluoride that goes into the municipal water is actually industrial toxic waste. It is not the sodium fluoride that goes into toothpaste. It is a waste product of fertilizer production. The waste is 26 percent hydrofluorosilicic acid and 74 percent wastewater that contains various amounts of heavy toxic metals. It is too toxic and too expensive to dispose of as hazardous waste, yet this same sludge (unchanged) is sent to cities all over the world to go into our drinking water. It is not purified, and the only ones policing this are the people who make it. Do you think that's a good idea? I spoke to a city worker who handles the fluoride treatment, and he told me that the fluoride in the air causes the stainless steel in the room to corrode! It is a corrosive toxic chemical.

Other health problems caused by fluoride include bone cancer (osteosarcoma), brain cell damage, muscle disorders, arthritis, bone fractures, cell death, blood disorders, infertility, and thyroid malfunction.

The Greater Boston Physicians for Social Responsibility reported, "Fluoride exposure, at levels that are experienced by a significant proportion of the population whose drinking water is fluoridated, may have adverse impacts on the developing brain."[20]

There is a branch of dentistry called holistic or biological dentistry that does not advocate the use of fluoride and mercury fillings. You can find more information at www.iamot.org, www.fluoridealert.org, and www.ewg.org.

What Should You Do?

You can go to government websites to find out how much fluoride is in your water. If it is being added, try to convince those in power to stop adding it. Get water that is processed by reverse osmosis or that is distilled and some type of filter to get rid of your water's fluoride. Don't use fluoride toothpaste. Use fluoride-free water for infant formula (and of course breast-feed first, when possible). Studies show that babies who are formula fed are getting exposed to higher levels of fluoride because tap water is used to make the formula; plus, there is fluoride in the formula. As the Academy of General Dentistry warns, "If you add fluoridated water to your infant's baby formula, you may be putting your child at risk of developing dental fluorosis."

Formula-fed babies can be exposed to two hundred times more fluoride than breastfed babies. Dr. Yolanda White (pediatrician) has said, "I diagnose dental fluorosis on average 5 times daily, but fluoride doesn't only affect teeth, it can potentially affect the brain and nervous system, kidneys, bones and other tissues in young children during their critical stages of organ development."

Healthy teeth come from the inside out and from good hygiene. We will look at hygiene further in chapter 8.

Aquatic Therapy

Water can also be therapeutic. After severe injuries, aquatic therapy can be very valuable if you can't put weight on a joint. Swimming is an excellent workout with very low likelihood of injury. It's not weight bearing, so it's not a good way to strengthen bones, but is a good place to start if you haven't been active for six months or more.

Taking baths is also good for the body. Put some Epsom salts and essential oils in the water. Light some candles and listen to some calming music for a great de-stressing time. Don't answer the phone, send the kids to bed, forget the e-mails, and just relax.

In the next chapter you will learn that eating certain foods will decrease your need to drink as much water as well as how to eat healthily for the rest of your life without dieting.

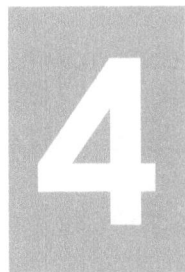

Food

> Then God said, "I give you every seed-bearing plant on the face of the whole earth and every tree that has fruit with seed in it. They will be yours for food ... everything that has the breath of life in it—I give every green plant for food."
>
> —Genesis 1:29–30

> Then after the flood God added the animals for food. "Everything that lives and moves will be food for you. Just as I gave you the green plants, I now give you everything. But you must not eat meat that has its lifeblood still in it."
>
> —Genesis 9:3–4

Never think of what you eat as a *diet*, because the name implies that the point is only to reach a weight-loss goal and that once you achieve it, you will go back to what you ate before. Instead, plan to change your lifestyle. It is best to make small changes, but the key to improving is to stick with it!

The information here is for everyone. Every human being has the same nutritional requirements. It doesn't matter what your gender is, what race, nationality, blood type, religion, or region of the world you are from. Every human being should eat the same types of foods, but of course we will have individual likes and dislikes. You may have certain sensitivities to some foods, but that is usually due to chemicals being on or in the food or some emotional stress response (more on that in chapter 10). There will be regional differences based on what grows locally or what is available, but the general principles will be the same. If you already have poor health and bowel disease, you may not be able to follow this advice as easily. Work with a licensed health-care provider for your specific needs. God has never said that some should be vegans, some should be carnivores, and some should only eat grains. He designed us to require the same nutrients. This is very clear: we are omnivores. There is no healthy plant source for vitamin B12; it comes from eggs and meats. There is no animal source for healthy fiber. We need both of these in the correct amounts.

Some people think that our blood types should dictate our eating, but according to Dr. James V. Linman, hematologist, "A single system may involve one or several antigens or blood group factors. An infinite number of combinations are possible and it seems that a person's precise blood type is as individually specific as are his fingerprints." As of 2005, twenty-two specific blood groups have been identified. It is not just the four that people used to think of (A, B, AB, and O).[21]

I know many Christians who think they can eat anything they want because of grace, unlike the Jewish people who follow strict dietary guidelines. I am going to boldly step out to say I disagree. I don't think Jesus abolished the old laws, because He followed them himself. He wasn't a slave to the laws, but He followed them because God had already established them for our benefit. There are two main places in Scripture that confuse this issue. In Matthew 15:11, Jesus says, "What goes into a man's mouth does not make him 'unclean,' but what comes out of his mouth, that is what makes him 'unclean.'" He goes on in verses 19 and 20 to say, "For out of the heart come evil thoughts, murder, adultery, sexual immorality, theft, lies, slander. These are what make a man 'unclean'; but eating with unwashed hands does not make him 'unclean.'" Here Jesus means *unclean* in a spiritual sense, as in "sinful." Eating certain foods doesn't make us sinful.

The other place that introduces confusion is Acts 10:11–29,

when Peter has a vision of all kinds of four-footed animals as well as reptiles of the earth and birds of the air. God tells Peter to kill and eat them. Peter doesn't want to eat these things because he has followed the Jewish laws regarding what animals to not eat: "I have never eaten anything impure or unclean." But God says, "Do not call anything impure that God has made clean." This happens *three* times. Then the Spirit tells Peter that three men are coming for him (non-Jews). In verse 28 Peter says, "God has shown me that I should not call any *man* impure or unclean" (emphasis mine). The vision is not about food; it is about people. Peter had associated gentiles with being unclean or sinful because they ate certain foods. As Jesus was teaching in Matthew 15, eating certain types of food is not sinful; it is our attitudes and actions that make us sinful. This doesn't mean we can eat anything we want without health consequences though.

Jesus said, "Do not think that I have come to abolish the Law or the Prophets; I have not come to abolish them but to fulfill them" (Matthew 5:17). In other words, the old law still stands, but we are to be accountable to Jesus (Holy Spirit)—not to human beings. John 14:21 records Jesus speaking to His disciples: "Whoever has my commands and obeys them, he is the one who loves me." We are to follow His commands so that we can be blessed with good health.

Lastly, according to 1 Corinthians 6:12–20, you are to "honor God with your body." Paul said, "Everything is permissible for me—but not everything is beneficial. Everything it permissible for me—but I will not be mastered by anything. Food for the stomach and the stomach for food." He also said, "Your body is a temple of the Holy Spirit." We don't *have* to follow the Old Testament laws, but we *should* because they will protect our health. I'm sure most people aren't going to eat rats, seagulls or crows, and for good reason: they often carry diseases. Other animals do too. Pigs and shellfish were designed to be natural cleaners and scavengers to clean up our lands and seas. If we eat those animals, we are eating toxins.

God loves us and gave us these warnings to protect us— not to hinder us or make life less pleasant. If we want to have the abundant life Jesus spoke of, we should seek to live how He lived. Just because God created pigs, rats, and shrimp doesn't mean they are there for us to eat. They have their purpose, and it is not to be food for people.

Somehow I have the sense that many people don't think the laws of nature apply to them when they follow Jesus. Sure, He can supernaturally heal us, but why would He when we continue to eat and live in a way that damages the temple? God calls us to be "set apart, holy, a royal priesthood." If our health problems are caused by ignoring these natural laws, God expects us to start following the healthy principles set out in the Bible before we will see healing. Ignoring the laws of good health is like ignoring the laws of physics. Sure, you could jump out of an airplane without a parachute and God *could* supernaturally put you safely on the ground, but what if He didn't? I think He wants us to use wisdom in all areas of life.

One of the biggest keys to improving your nutritional habits is to add healthy changes before taking away any unhealthy foods. Psychologically this is easier to do. Whenever we are told we can't do something, we almost automatically go and do it.

The first step is to determine your goals. If your goal is to lose weight, get a slim waist, bigger biceps, or fewer chins, you may end up causing yourself more harm. *Make improving your health the goal.* If you focus on getting healthy, weight loss, better body image, and more energy will follow.

The second step is to add fresh, raw fruits and vegetables to your diet. As God said in Genesis 1, we are to eat fruits and vegetables. We were vegetarians for several generations, but after the great flood that changed. It doesn't matter if you can find studies showing the benefits of being a vegetarian; God said to eat animals. According to Genesis, the first people were vegetarians, but after the flood that changed. In Genesis 9:2–3, God gives the fish and says that "everything that lives and moves will be food for you. Just as I gave you the green plants ..." Often when people become vegetarian, they cut out more of the unhealthy foods and, of course, benefit from this change, but eating animals is necessary for getting enough protein, minerals (iron, calcium, and zinc), saturated fats, vitamin D, and vitamin B12.[22] I realize that with artificial supplementation people can get enough of these nutrients; however, that isn't as healthy as getting it from nature.

I like Dr. James Chestnut's catch phrase: "Fresh Fibre First."[23] Fresh means uncooked, fibre means vegetable or fruit, and first means before you eat anything else. Whether it's a meal or a snack, always have fresh fibre first. Eating raw vegetables and fruits is better than cooked, canned, or frozen. Fresh vegetables retain the enzymes and nutrients so you get more vitamins and minerals. Plus, it makes it easier for your body to digest any other food you might be eating. Vegetables and fruits are high in fiber, so they help to fill us up with relatively low calories. If you were to eat a meal-sized salad at every meal, I guarantee you would get healthier. Since vegetables and fruits are low in calories, they make us feel full. We need other foods in addition, which I will discuss in a moment. It is more beneficial to have the vegetables or fruit first for several reasons. Number one, it ensures that we actually eat them. Many people say that they will have their salad after they eat other foods first, but often they are then too full. By eating a salad first, there is no missing out. Second, if you eat anything after your fresh fiber that is not healthy, you will eat less of it because your stomach will already be full of healthy foods. Finally, eating fiber-rich foods first helps with eliminating wastes through the colon.

Vegetables and fruits should be the majority of the calories we eat daily. Aim for 40 percent of your total daily calories from fruits and vegetables.

Many people wonder why we shouldn't just eat more grains to get more fiber. Vegetables and fruits by far outweigh grains when it comes to fiber, as you can see in Figure 3.1.

Figure 3.1 Total Fibre (Grams) per 1,000-Calorie Serving[24]

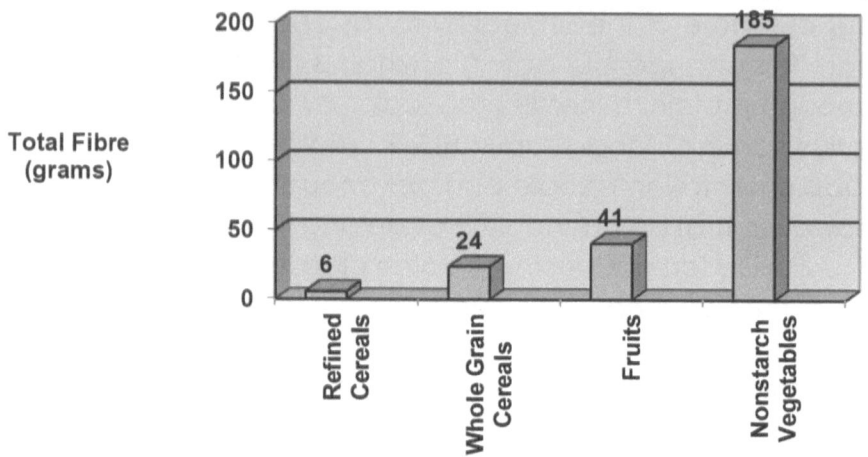

Good Carbs, Bad Carbs

There has been a huge surge in diet books talking about low-carb diets. We need carbohydrates, but there are good ones and there are bad ones. Good carbs are found in vegetables and fruits and some grains. Bad carbs are found in processed or sugary junk foods. Simple carbs are easily converted into sugar, and then they enter the bloodstream to create havoc with our insulin levels. Big spikes in insulin lead to big drops in energy. High sugar loads also lead to increased fat storage. In other words, consuming too many bad carbs leads to increased body fat levels. As you can see from Figure 3.1, refined cereals are low in fibre, which leads to a greater increase in blood sugar levels.

Good carbs are lower on the glycemic index, which is a measure of how much sugar is in a food. The bad carbs listed below are in the high-glycemic range, meaning they raise blood sugars quite quickly. It might surprise you that sweet potatoes and yams, even though they taste sweeter than white potatoes, are actually quite a bit lower on the glycemic index.[25]

Figure 3.2 Comparisons of Good Carbohydrates and Bad Carbohydrates

Good Carbohydrates	Bad Carbohydrates
Vegetables Fruits Sprouted seeds (includes buckwheat) Whole sprouted grains (oatmeal, wild and brown rice, millet, barley, quinoa, spelt) Sprouted beans	Refined sugars (includes liquid sugars, soft drinks, corn syrup) Artificial sugars (Aspartame, Saccharin, etc.) Refined cereals (Cheerios, corn flakes, Froot Loops, etc.) Chips and other junk foods White bread White rice Skim milk, other non-fat dairy Candy

What do vegetarian zombies eat? Grains! If you don't want to feel like a zombie, eat good carbs. Remember, I didn't say we couldn't have the bad carbs, because then automatically that's what we would want to eat. Have your healthy carbs first, and then a small amount of unhealthy carbs won't be so bad. Or better yet, limit your unhealthy food choices to one day per week. That's what I do. I have my one "junk food day." I eat whatever I want on the unhealthy list and don't feel bad about it because I am eating healthy the rest of the week. That doesn't mean you should go crazy and gorge yourself silly. For example, we don't eat unhealthy desserts during the week, only on our junk food day. If you want dessert more often, have some fruit. A bowl of strawberries or a fruit salad is really nice.

There is a huge problem today with people being addicted to sugar. I would guess that it is the number one addiction in the world (caffeine would be number two). More and more people every year are damaging their pancreas to the point of developing type 2 diabetes, which is almost 100 percent caused by unhealthy choices. Type 2 diabetes is almost completely preventable and reversible if caught soon enough.

According to the Canadian Diabetes Association, there are 285 million people worldwide with diabetes. Today one out of every three people is expected to develop diabetes! Diabetes leads to obesity, cardiac disease, blindness, stroke, amputation of limbs, and shortened life span. As an individual with diabetes, expect to pay up to $15,000 per year in extra healthcare costs. In ten years diabetes is expected to cost Canadian healthcare $17 billion a year![26] In the US, in the year 2007 alone, diabetes cost $174 billion![27] Further, the costs are escalating every year. Here is how you help solve the global economic crisis: Improve your health, because we are all suffering for it. Remember, this is a problem that is almost 100 percent preventable. All it takes is some lifestyle changes, and you will feel better, look better, and have more energy to devote to your Father, your family, and your friends.

When sugar levels are high in the bloodstream, insulin levels go up. High insulin levels prevent us from converting fats into energy. Instead, our bodies use the sugars in the blood to make the energy they need, and then they store any leftover sugar as fat. For years people have been told that to lose fat they needed to eat less fat because fat has fewer calories per gram than carbohydrates. This is true; however, that's not how it works in our bodies. To lose body fat a person must decrease simple (bad) carbohydrates.

Good carbs lead to fat loss. Bad carbs lead to fat gain.

High insulin levels also increase stress hormones, which interfere with our immune system. Our bodies can no longer effectively fight foreign invaders or cancer cells when our immune systems are down. A blood sugar level of 120 limits the immune system (phagocytic index) by 75 percent! One saltine cracker causes blood sugar to spike to between one hundred and 150 for five to six hours. This means that for five to six hours after eating a saltine or any other high simple carbohydrate (high glycemic) food, our ability to destroy harmful viruses, bacteria, cancer, and other pathogens is decreased by 75 percent. The odds are pretty good that a person will get sick who might not otherwise have done so in the several hours after consuming bad carbs.

Here's how it usually goes in the real world. You go to a birthday party (Christmas party, staff party, wedding, Halloween party, etc.), and there's someone there who says he has a cold. You're feeling fine and think nothing of it. The food is good, you eat too much, the desserts are divine, and you drink something sugary (pop, juice, wine, etc.). You feel good. The next day or two days later you don't feel so good. It was so-and-so's fault: "He gave me his cold." Your family who attended the same function also gets the same symptoms (which are your body's detoxifying reaction to get you healthier), and you are convinced that the germs were just passed around. Sure, you may have been exposed to something by someone, but your immune system couldn't fight it because the sugar levels caused high insulin levels, leading to decreased immune function. Sound familiar? Viruses, bacteria, and all other microscopic organisms were all created at the same time, thousands of years ago, along with all the other animals (Genesis 1). Our immune system has been adapting and killing them off ever since.

Try this next time you go to one of those functions. Eat fresh fiber first (raw vegetables, salad), and put healthy oil on it (flax, olive, hemp, fish oil). Drink water. Eat lean, healthy meats (if available). Try fish, wild game, or grass-fed beef—not hot dogs. Eat cooked vegetables. Skip the white pasta. Have fruit for dessert. Encourage your family to eat all the junk. Go talk to someone who claims to be sick. Get to bed at a good hour. For the following couple of days, continue to eat well, exercise, and spend time in prayer and reading the Bible. See how *you* feel. See how *your family* feels.

You might still get sick if you haven't been living well for years, but if you change your choices, you will get healthier and notice the difference. And remember that you might feel worse at times, even if your cellular health has improved. Health is not about feelings but function, so if your body is functioning properly, you will get symptoms when it is detoxifying or killing infectious organisms.

Our Daily Bread

Many sources are coming down hard on gluten, breads, and other grains because there is a large increase in the number of people who have a problem digesting them. Let me first tell you what God says, and then I will explain why grains can still be problematic.

In Genesis 41 Joseph tells Pharaoh the meaning of his dreams about cows and grain. Joseph advises Pharaoh to store up enough grain to last for seven years of famine. Sure enough, there is enough grain to sustain Egypt for seven years. God doesn't tell him to store up carrots or apples; He tells him to store up grain.

Exodus 12:17 says, "Celebrate the Feast of Unleavened Bread ... as a lasting ordinance for the generations to come." It is pretty clear that this feast is to carry on indefinitely. And in the New Testament Jesus says, "Give us this day our daily bread," which is where we get the Lord's Prayer from.

In John 21:9 Jesus feeds His disciples a breakfast of fish and bread. This is His last recorded meal with them. Most people aren't going to eat fish and bread for breakfast, but why not? It's a whole lot healthier for us than Cheerios or some other typical breakfast.

Of course we can't forget Communion (Passover): the bread and the cup. Jesus even called himself the "bread of life."

If wheat is so bad, why is it mentioned so often and given

such significance in the Bible? It's not bad, but the Enemy wants to go against anything good, so of course he will attack the "bread of life."

Bread and grains are not the problem; they were designed for us to eat. The problem is the pesticides, genetically modified crops, preservatives, and other chemicals that poison the grain crops. Then the grains are overly refined and bleached, making them unhealthy. Think of commercial breads and flours like potato chips. Potatoes are healthy, but potato chips are not.

Eat organic *sprouted* whole grains, not white bread, white pasta, or white flour. Years ago bread was made from spouted whole grains, freshly ground. Also, sprouted grains don't contain the same levels of phytic acid. When a grain is sprouted it essentially becomes a vegetable, which changes its nutritional value. The world has a sneaky way of taking something good and messing it up.

The other reason why so many are sensitive to gluten is the use of vaccines and antibiotics during childhood. Vaccines lead to food allergies and sensitivities in about 50 percent of all vaccinated people. Also, many children are fed formula instead of breast milk, which can lead to a leaky gut. Introducing foreign proteins to the digestive system too soon causes large and improperly digested protein molecules to pass from the gut into the bloodstream, causing an immune reaction. This later gives rise to sensitivities and allergies. So grains are not the enemy; modern medicine and agribusiness are.

Most people usually eat way too many grains anyway. Stick with no more than two servings per day. Fruits and vegetables are far more nutritious, so eat more salads and fewer sandwiches.

Acidic Foods

Some foods cause our bodies to become acidic. Normally our pH level should be around 7.4, which is slightly alkaline.

However, certain foods will cause our blood to become more acidic, which then causes our bodies to have to compensate by taking calcium out of our bones to neutralize the acidity. If this process goes on too long or if we are not getting enough calcium, we end up with a calcium deficiency, which starts to cause weakened bones, brittle nails and hair, muscle cramps, convulsions, numbness and tingling in the hands and feet, and abnormal heart rhythms that could lead to death if severe.[28]

Our innate intelligence wants to keep our blood pH optimal; otherwise, we will die. If it has to sacrifice our bones to keep us alive, it will. Our brain will always do what is best for us under the circumstances.

Acidity in our bodies also weakens the immune system; allows cancer cells to grow; allows parasites, yeasts, and other pathogenic microorganisms to grow; and leads to other diseases.

Foods that are acidic include all those listed in the bad carbs table: refined grains, bad fats, sugars, and animal products, such as meat and dairy. Vegetables and fruits are alkaline and thereby neutralize the acidity. We need a balance of both; being too alkaline is not healthy either. Try to get most of your foods from the alkaline side to keep the proper pH level in the body.

You can test you body's pH with a simple saliva or urinary test strip that is available at most health food stores, or you can order it online. On the following pages I have included a chart with some common foods and their pH or acidity values.

Figure 3.3: The Acid/Alkaline Values of Various Foods[29]

Foods	Most Acidic (pH 6 to 6.6)
Vegetables, beans, legumes	Peanut butter, soybeans
Fruits	Dried fruit, olives, pickles, canned fruit, jam, jelly
Seasonings, spices, herbs	MSG, black pepper, ketchup, mayonnaise, soy sauce

Foods	Most Acidic (pH 6 to 6.6)
Beverages	Alcohol, soft drinks, coffee with milk and sugar
Grains, cereals	Barley, cakes, cookies, pastries, oats, rye, white flour, white rice
Nuts, seeds, oils	Trans fats, pistachio, cashew, pecan, walnut
Meats, fish, fowl	Beef, lobster, chicken, veal, lamb, pork
Dairy, eggs	Processed cheese, soy cheese, ice cream, eggs
Sweeteners	Artificial sweeteners, corn syrup, fructose, sugar, high-fructose corn syrup
Vinegar	White vinegar, balsamic

Neutral (pH 6.8 to 7.2)	Most Alkaline (pH 7.4 to 8)
Corn, lentils, beans, green peas, beets, tomatoes, lettuce, potatoes, squash	Peppers, celery, spinach, carrot, asparagus, yams, kale, broccoli, garlic, onion,
Grapes, blueberry, strawberry, papaya, blackberry, banana, date, fig	Apple, avocado, cucumber, citrus, pear, melons, cherry, raspberry, raisin, mango
Tahini, carob, cocoa, most herbs, curry, mustard	Cinnamon, ginger, dill, mint, sea salt, cayenne, basil, oregano, parsley, tumeric
Rice milk, black coffee, black tea, dry red wine	Ozonated water, aloe vera, teas (green, ginger, rooibos)
Brown & basmati rice, wheat, buckwheat, quinoa, spelt, millet, whole grains	

Neutral (pH 6.8 to 7.2)	Most Alkaline (pH 7.4 to 8)
Hemp seed, canola, pine, hazelnut, flaxseed, coconut	Olive oil, Brazil nut, pumpkin seeds, almonds
Cod liver oil, fish, turkey, wild duck, venison	Wild fish
Yogurt, cream, butter, goat cheese, goat milk	Whey protein, human breast milk
Honey, stevia, maple syrup, brown rice syrup	Unsulfured blackstrap molasses
Rice vinegar	Apple cider vinegar

Juicing

Juicing raw vegetables is the best way to get your vitamins. In fact, many books have been written on juicing as a way to detoxify and heal cancer.[30] Juicing releases many nutrients that chewing doesn't, and juicing is not going to add the preservatives and other fillers that a multivitamin pill will. Juicing keeps the vitamins and enzymes vital, and freshly made juice is easy to digest. The downside of juicing is that the fiber is not used, but you can save it to add to foods like salads or to use as compost for a garden.

Good Fats, Bad Fats

There has been a lot of talk over the last few years about the different kinds of fats and which ones are good for us and which ones make us sick. We need fat in order to be healthy. In other words, low-fat diets are *not* healthy. A person might lose some short-term weight, but low-fat intake is not really sustainable will eventually lead to the person gaining all the lost weight back and then some. In 1953 Ancel Keys (an American scientist) decided that eating too much fat would make people fat. He made a diagram showing the correlation between fat consumption and dying from heart disease in six countries, which he carefully selected out of twenty-two countries that had the data available. The diagram showed that the more fat that people consumed, the higher the number of deaths from heart disease. However, when the data from the other sixteen countries was added back in, the correlation disappeared. In other words, there was and still is no good evidence to support this claim, yet many are still teaching it. Ever since this idea was introduced, the rates of obesity have been increasing, as have the rates of heart disease and cancer.[31]

The problem is that there *are* healthy fats and unhealthy fats, so it's a bit confusing. We need to get around 30 percent of our daily calories from healthy fats. For someone eating 2,500 calories per day, that would be 825 calories from fats. That would work out to around ninety-two grams of fat per day. Don't worry; you don't have to count calories to be healthy, but you do need to watch your portion sizes.

Figure 3.4 Table of Good Fats and Bad Fats

Good Fats	Bad Fats
Cold-water fish	Peanuts
Flaxseed oil	Cottonseed oil
Hemp seed oil	Sunflower oil
Olive oil	Grape seed oil
Coconut oil	Safflower oil
Walnuts and almonds	Canola oil
Avocado	All hydrogenated fats
Organic meats, chicken,	Margarine
Turkey, duck	Butter substitutes
Wild game meats	Shell fish
Organic butter	
Whole eggs	

Many people have been led to believe that eating fats causes fat gain. It's not true! We need to eat fat, just not the bad fats. In fact, if we don't get enough fat we will die. Every cell in our bodies needs and contains fats. When we don't get enough fats, our bodies have to sacrifice some tissues to save the vital organs. Usually the first places that suffer are the joints, hair, and skin. They are not as important as our hearts, brains, and livers in keeping us alive. That's why many skin conditions improve when a person starts eating more good fats.

Have you ever noticed that the dog food commercials talk about how shiny the coat of a dog is from eating their brand of food? Good health comes from the inside.

When we eat the right kinds of fats we feel better, look better, and get healthier. Consuming good fat leads us to burn fat, and consuming bad fat leads us to gain fat. In order to lose fat, you just might need to eat more good fats.

Frying

Some healthy fats become unhealthy when you heat them up. These are the healthy fats you can fry with: coconut, walnut, almond, and butter. Other healthy fats, such as hemp seed and olive oil, become unhealthy when you heat them up too much. Use these at lower temperatures only.

A License to Krill

Right now krill oil is being touted as the best source of omega-3 fatty acids. There are two main types of omega-3 essential fats: DHA and EPA. Krill oil is high in one type, DHA, whereas fish oil is high in DHA and EPA. Flax oil contains neither. It has a different omega-3 that our bodies can use to convert to one type of omega-3, called ALA. Many of the cold-water fish will eat krill, which is a very small shrimp-like creature that whales also eat. Humans have never eaten krill, but we do eat the fish that eat krill. When we eat the fish, we enjoy the health benefits. However, our bodies were not designed to eat krill; it is fish food. Even though krill does contain healthy oil, it's not for people. It's just marketing. Because fish oil has been around for years, it's time to give people "the latest and greatest."

I don't know if you've noticed, but about every six to twelve months a new "super food" comes out that you just have to have. There was mangosteen, then goji berries, then pomegranates, and then acai berries. It is all about marketing. God said all plants and seeds are good. They all have benefits, so get a variety. Don't be fooled by a network marketing company into thinking they have the answer to everyone's health problems. Turning everything into juice makes it unhealthy unless you make it fresh daily. Plus, in order to keep the juice from going bad, preservatives are added (toxins).

So forget the hype. Get your nutrients the way God intended, in their least processed form. Don't buy into the marketing. If you want krill, get krill, but don't be fooled into thinking that it is better.

Inflammatory Foods

Some foods cause inflammation in the body—not the healthy kind of inflammation that is the first stage in healing but high levels that are unhealthy. This is due to eating high levels of omega-6 fats, which are listed in the bad fats column. High levels of bad fats actually cause inflammatory diseases, such as arthritis, inflammatory bowel syndrome, eczema, kidney disease, liver disease, and others. Simply by adding the good fats and eliminating the bad fats, you can reverse or prevent these problems.

Another source of inflammation is MSG (monosodium glutamate). It is found in almost every food that has flavours added.MSG causes over stimulation of the brain, addiction to foods, inflammation, weight gain and eventually brain cell death. Avoid MSG as much as you can.

Good Protein, Bad Protein

Table 3.5 Comparison of Good Protein Sources and Bad Protein Sources

Good Proteins	Bad Proteins
Wild fish (with fins and scales)	Farmed fish
Wild game (moose, bison, deer, etc.)	Shellfish (crab, shrimp)
Organic free-range chicken and turkey, pheasant, grouse, duck	Any type of fish that does not have fins and scales (shark, dolphin, porpoise)
Organic free-range eggs	Feedlot beef
Organic, free-range beef, lamb, goat	Chicken, turkey
Canned wild fish	Non-organic eggs
Skip jack tuna	Albacore and yellowfin tuna
Organic non-pasteurized dairy (milk, cream, yogurt, cheese)	Pasteurized non-organic dairy
Organic goat's milk, cheese, yogurt	Processed meats (salami, sausage, pepperoni, hot dog, etc.)
Locust, katydid, cricket, or grasshopper	Pork (ham, bacon, etc.)
Homemade organic sausage made with any of the healthy meats	Rodents (rat, weasel, etc.)
	Reptiles (lizard, snake, gecko, chameleon, etc.)
	Any animal that chews grass but does not have a split hoof (rabbit, camel, badger)
	Types of flying insect and bat
	Birds of prey (owl, eagle, vulture, raven, crow, hawk, gull, stork heron, cormorant)

*see Leviticus chapter 11

The biggest factor in what makes an animal healthy or not is what it eats (just like us). If you eat an animal that was fed grass sprayed with pesticides or given steroids, hormones, or antibiotics, then you are eating pesticides, steroids, and hormones. Pesticides are toxic chemicals that cause cancer. Since the pesticides bioaccumulate over time, meat eaters ingest higher levels of toxins than vegans, so research shows that vegans generally have lower rates of cancers. But it's not the fact that vegans are avoiding meats that helps prevent cancers; it is the fact that they are avoiding toxins. We need the meat, not the chemicals, so choose your food sources wisely.

Avoid Dangerous Cookware

A recent study showed that chemicals found commonly in non-stick cookware are linked to thyroid disease. Perfluoroctanoic acid (PFOA) and perfluoroctane sulphonate (PFOS) in small amounts over time can lead to low thyroid hormone levels.[32] Low thyroid levels are linked to high blood pressure, abnormal heart rate, weight gain, decreased immune function, poor mental health (depression, poor memory), skin disorders, slow reflexes, infertility, and abnormally low body temperature.[33] Also, avoid aluminum cookware, as it also has potentially deadly consequences with use over time.

Use safe cookware, such as cast iron, stainless steel, or stoneware. It's not as easy to clean, and it can be sticky, but your health is on the line. There are some safe oils for frying with: organic butter, coconut oil, sesame oil, almond oil, and walnut oil. Don't use flax, hemp, or olive oil for frying at higher temperatures because it changes the oil into an unhealthy form.

Try not to overeat, even if it is healthy food. Many people become addicted to food. They use it as a comforter. They eat when they are happy, sad, scared, or depressed or for any number of other reasons. Let God be your comfort. It's important to use self-control, "for a man is a slave to whatever has mastered him" (2 Peter 2:19). Don't let food master you; see it as a tool to be used to bring about good health.

Fasting or Cleansing

There are different kinds of fasts listed in the Bible for different reasons, so your goals will dictate what kind of fast is best. Probably the easiest fast to start with is given in Daniel 1. Daniel, Hanniah, Mishael, and Azariah ate nothing but vegetables and water for ten days. They consumed no meats, no dairy, no wheat or other grains (corn), no juice, no coffee, and no chocolate. Verse 15 says, "At the end of the ten days they looked healthier and better nourished than any of the young men you ate the royal food." Not only were they now healthier, "to these four young men God gave knowledge and understating of all kinds of literature and learning. And Daniel could understand visions and dreams of all kinds" (Daniel 1:17). The King "found them ten times better than all the magicians and enchanters in his whole kingdom" (Daniel 1: 20).

I don't know if God will grant you all of these blessings, but have faith that He will bless you if you follow His ways. If nothing else, the ten-day fast will improve your physical health. By eating only vegetables (soups, salads, beans), your body will be able to cleanse.

Juice fasting is another great way to cleanse yourself of physical and spiritual toxins. If you are being controlled by food (emotional eating, overeating, or unhealthy eating), you need to take control of your food. Drinking only juices for three days will allow you to bring yourself under control. You can do this by just drinking fresh homemade vegetable and fruit juices. Try to use more vegetables than fruits to lower your sugar intake and increase your vitamin intake.

Another useful juice technique is one called the Master Cleanse® or lemon juice fast.[34] In this fast, you would combine two tablespoons of maple syrup with two tablespoons of fresh lemon juice and a pinch of cayenne pepper in a large glass of pure water. Every time you get hungry, you drink the lemon drink. This can easily be followed for three days. Don't eat anything else except for herbal tea or pure water.

It is a good idea to ease into a fast. Start by decreasing your food intake a day or two before you start the fast. Decrease any unhealthy foods and drink more water.

There are common pitfalls during a fast that cause many to stumble. The most common one is being around others who are eating. Eating is social, and it is hard to be the only one not eating. If you can, fast with someone else in your home. The second most common pitfall is the detoxifying process that happens. Expect to feel worse the first or second day. Not eating gives your body the ability to cleanse or detoxify. The toxins are then eliminated, but you will feel worse in the process. Remind yourself that this is a good thing. You will feel better and be healthier by the third day.

During the fast, spend the time you normally would on meal preparation, eating, and cleaning up on spiritual disciplines. Pray, meditate, read the Bible, practice healthy breathing, take a detox bath, or go on a nice walk.

Coming out of a fast is more important than before or during the fast. On the morning of the "breakfast," start by drinking some water followed by a healthy juice. Orange juice seems to work well, just not too concentrated. Depending on how long you have been fasting, you might just have juice for breakfast. Follow this up with fruit and vegetable smoothies, vegetable broths, and soups. Do not eat any grains, dairy, or meats. On day two after the fast, you can add in salads, cooked vegetables, nuts, seeds, and small amounts of yogurt (plain only). Day three you can add in small amounts of healthy meats, grains, and dairy. Remember to keep the meals small and mostly vegetables. Then keep it going!

Genetically Modified Organisms (GMOs)

The name "genetically modified organism" basically says it all. These are human-manipulated plants that big corporations claim will solve all our problems. But beware of the wolf in sheep's clothing. If God didn't create it, we aren't designed to digest it. Humans can *never* improve on God's creation.

Big drug companies design these products to be resistant to pesticides so they can spray them like crazy and not kill the plants. So people end up ingesting higher levels of toxic chemicals.

GMO tomatoes might look nicer, taste sweeter, and be more disease resilient but who cares if they cause cancer, other diseases, or death? In one study done on FLAVR SAVR™ tomatoes, by the company that engineered them, seven out of forty rats fed these tomatoes died within two weeks. They didn't even bother to investigate why the rats mysteriously died.[35]

Genetically modified (GM) foods have been shown to cause kidney, liver, and stomach diseases; cancer; inflammatory bowel diseases; miscarriages; stillbirths; and autoimmune disorders, such as ALS and rheumatoid arthritis.

In order to genetically modify a plant, genes are attached to *viruses* that carry the genes into the plant. This is foolish and dangerous, so avoid all GM foods. The most commonly GM crops are tomatoes, potatoes, rice, corn, peas, soybeans, and cotton. There is much more information available; if you want to learn more, go to www.biointegrity.org.

We and our children are the guinea pigs, and the corporations are making huge profits. Sixty percent of all processed foods in North America now contain GMOs. Greater than 90 percent of all soy, canola, and sugar beets (high-fructose corn syrup) produced in America are GM.

Zambia, Venezuela, Hungary, and most European countries have already banned the import of GM foods. If a country as poor and needy as Zambia is saying, "We would rather starve than eat your GM foods," that says a lot.

You can identify GM produce by the PLU (price look up) code sticker on the item. All GM foods start with the number eight and are followed by four other numbers. For example, a genetically engineered tomato would be 84805. A regular non-organic, non-GM tomato would be 4805.

Organic produce PLU codes start with the number nine. For example, an organic banana would be 94011 whereas a non-organic, but not GM banana would be 4011.[36]

Regular produce has only four numbers, but it will contain pesticides and will not have been grown with healthy practices.

Don't be left in the dark: read the labels. Avoid all soy, canola, corn, and sugar that are not certified organic. That means soymilk, soybeans, soy oil, soy sauce, teriyaki (contains soy), canola oil, corn oil, corn chips, corn meal, sugar, liquid sugar, HFCS (high-fructose corn syrup), and sugar beets. The two most common oils in products today are soy and canola. These are found in salad dressing, mayonnaise, soups, sauces, prepared foods, snack foods, and junk foods. Soy is added as a filler to lunch meats, hamburgers, hot dogs, and other processed foods. Soy and canola oils are in breads, cakes, crackers, and cookies.

Shopping today is like going into battle; if you are not prepared (educated), you will lose.

Another issue to consider is the amount of animal products that you eat. The pancreas makes enzymes that enable our bodies to digest food. It is also responsible for destroying cancer cells. If a person is eating animal products all day, the pancreas is using its energy to digest food and not spending any time killing cancer cells. Natural cancer treatment experts advise cancer patients to avoid eating meat to give the pancreas time to kill the cancer. If you don't have cancer but are trying to prevent it, then eat only two consecutive meals that contain animal products (fat or protein). For example, only eat animal products at breakfast and lunch or at lunch and dinner.

Generally it is better to eat more in the beginning of the day and less toward the end of the day. Jesus served His disciples a meal of fish and bread for breakfast the last time He saw them on Earth in John 21:9. There is nothing wrong with eating fish for breakfast. It's probably not the tradition in your home, but there is no reason you couldn't do it. Or have a salad for breakfast, and then at lunch time you could have some organic meat. Or have eggs at breakfast and fish at lunch. Then dinner could be a vegan meal (no dairy, meat, or other animal products). You could have nuts, seeds, or beans in the evening for protein.

Supplements

Many people today take supplements that are not necessary. Human beings have survived for thousands of years without taking artificial nutrients. The argument for supplements is that the soil is depleted or that it is just too hard to get all you need from food today. The reality is that eating fresh fruits and vegetables all year is possible and actually easier than it was one hundred years ago. Today we can eat food from around the world all year long. In the past a person could only eat fresh during the growing season; if you lived in a climate with a real winter, your options were limited. Most people learned to can or preserve food. This is better than nothing, but it is not as beneficial as fresh food.

Even if you eat fresh and organic foods, there are still a few areas that you could be deficient in. Therefore I do recommend that you take a couple of supplements for wellness. The first and most important is omega-3 oil. Omega-3, as mentioned earlier, is an essential fat that all our cells need for proper function, and it is deficient in most diets. You would have to be eating fish twice a day to get enough. Cold-water fish is the best source of omega-3s, but be sure to get a good-quality fish that is guaranteed to be mercury free. A good rule of thumb for omega-3s is a quarter teaspoon for every twenty pounds of body weight. That applies to kids and adults.

Another supplement to consider is one that contains probiotics. Probiotics are healthy bacteria (more on that in chapter 11) that help our bodies digest food and kill unhealthy bacteria. Most people need these because of the antibiotics in our world today.

As mentioned in chapter 1, we need vitamin D to be healthy. From October to April in the northern areas mentioned in chapter 1, be sure to supplement with vitamin D. A good rule of thumb is to take five hundred international units for every fifty pounds of body weight. Children under fifty pounds should get five hundred international units per day, and adults over two hundred pounds need 2000 international units per day.

If you want a good multivitamin, buy a juicer and make your own, as discussed previously. Or, if that's not viable at this time, Douglas Laboratories makes a product called Organic Greens and Reds, which is organic green and red vegetables and fruits that have been juiced and then dehydrated. Each small scoop contains the nutrients of three to four servings of fruit and vegetables. Of course, it's better to get natural-state nutrients than those that have been turned into a pill or a powder.

Do *not* buy supplements from Costco, Wal-Mart, or any drug stores, as you will most likely be buying toxins as well as your supplement. Buy supplements from a licensed natural health practitioner because such individuals are responsible for the products they sell and therefore usually sell better products. Your health is valuable, so don't go cheap on food or supplements. Buy high-quality food and save money on other things. You are worth it, and in the end it will save you money on doctor's bills.

Of course if you are eating, you should also be moving. Exercise is the focus of the next chapter; how often and how much should you exercise?

Exercise

> For physical training is of some value, but godli-
> ness has value for all things, holding promise for
> both the present life and the life to come.
>
> > -1 Timothy 4:8

How much exercise does a person need, and how often should one exercise to be healthy? The short answer is you need to exercise six days per week to be healthy. Exodus 20:10 says, "The seventh day is a day of rest dedicated to the Lord your God." And Exodus 23:12 reinforces this by stating, "Work for six days and rest on the seventh ..."

No one can go without taking a break, so take a break one day per week so that you can be refreshed. This does not mean you lie around all Saturday or Sunday (or whichever day is your Sabbath). You can be active but not exercising or working. A leisurely Sunday stroll can be refreshing for many; just don't turn it into an exercise session. Playing with your children or grandchildren can be exercise or fun, depending on your fitness level.

If you are like most people, your challenge is that you need to exercise more. Notice God said to rest one day, not six days a week. Exercise is a vital nutrient to our health. It is the way our bodies are designed. Without weekly exercise, our bodies start to deteriorate. Unlike human-made objects that break down with use, our divinely designed bodies *improve* with use! It is not too much activity that leads to osteoporosis, heart attacks, obesity, diabetes, cancer, and arthritis, but inactivity.

All of these problems can be prevented by following the principles laid out in this book.

Many people are confused about the difference between being active and exercising. All day in my practice I am active, but that's not exercise. I've worn a pedometer to see how far I walk in a day, and it's around 11 kilometers (6.5 miles). If I were four hundred pounds and sedentary, that would be considered exercise. *Exercise* is defined as "work over time that is of limited duration." Since my body has adapted to that level of activity, it is no longer exercise. It could be argued that a heavy-duty mechanic gets a lot of exercise in a day. He or she is most likely only doing one type of exercise: strengthening. However, there are four types of exercise a person needs to perform to be healthy. The good news for the mechanic is that he or she would not need to make time to do strengthening exercises, but the other three are still necessary.

The time of day to exercise depends on the type of exercise you are doing. For certain types of exercise, it doesn't matter as long as you don't exercise right before you plan to go to bed, as you will find it harder to fall asleep. I prefer to exercise early in the morning. It's a great way to start the day, and I have found that if I don't exercise in the morning, I'm not likely to find the time to do it later. By exercising in the morning, I don't miss out on time with my family.

A person can worship God through exercise. 1 Timothy 4:8 says, "For physical training is of some value, but godliness has value for all things, holding promise for both the present life and for the life to come." Invite God to join you as you walk alongside a bubbling creek or on a treadmill at home. You can go on prayer walks and accomplish physical training that is of *some value* while learning godliness, which has *more value*, at the same time. The interests and activities that you enjoy were given to you by God. He will enjoy spending time with you doing the things you like to do. It is easier to sense God's presence outside, so as much as possible do your exercise outside. Plus, you will also get the benefit of cleaner air and sunlight. "What does the Lord require of you? To act justly, and to love mercy and to *walk* humbly with your God" (Micah 6:8, emphasis mine).

There are four types of exercise you need to perform to be healthy: cardiovascular, strengthening, stretching, and postural.

Cardiovascular

This is also called aerobic exercise because the need for oxygen increases. The easiest and most cost effective way to get you aerobic exercise is through walking. It has to be more than a casual jaunt. It should be at a pace that causes your heart rate to go up and your breathing rate to increase. In other words, your goal should be brisk walking.

You need to get sixty minutes of aerobic exercise six days per week. Even getting thirty minutes of brisk walking six days per week will decrease your likelihood of getting cancer and heart disease by up to 50 percent![37] This can be broken down into two thirty-minute sessions. If you are just starting to exercise, you might have to start at fifteen minutes once per day and then go to two times per day. After you can do that, start adding more time. When you can perform the exercise without stopping for sixty minutes per day, then you can increase your intensity. So if you were walking, you would start interspersing jogging with your walking. Be sure to consult a licensed doctor of chiropractic before starting your exercise program so that you don't do something that could cause you damage.

Other examples of cardiovascular exercise include my favorite, Olympic rowing (sculling), swimming, cross country skiing, gymnastics, cycling, hiking, martial arts, team sports (such as soccer and basketball), cross training, and fitness classes (kickboxing, aquatic fitness, CrossFit, and low-impact aerobics). There are many others, so find something you enjoy.

Exercise should be enjoyable. If you are a social person, do social exercise. If you are more of an introverted person, a solo sport might be better for you. Most people are more likely to stick with an exercise program if they have a partner or group that holds them accountable and asks why they missed a workout, but most of all it should be fun. Most adults forget that when we were kids we called exercise "play." We would run around, climb on monkey bars, play tag, and have a great time, all the while not realizing that we were exercising. So play.

Strengthening

There are dozens of different strength-training regimes available, so I am just going to give some general guidelines. Unlike cardiovascular exercise, strengthening or anaerobic exercises only need to be performed two or three times per week. Twice a week is sufficient for beginners, and three times per week is sufficient when you are more advanced.

Olympic and power lifting are great ways to improve your strength while maintaining flexibility. Gymnastic movements are also great for strength, and CrossFit workouts have a combination of all three.

It's best to work out the entire body at each session. Whenever possible, perform exercises that use more body parts rather than isolating muscles. Isolation exercises will lead to strength gains, but they lead to functionally weak and unbalanced muscles also. By functionally weak, I mean that the bicep may be strong at doing bicep curls, but if a person then goes to play baseball he or she could actually endure a bicep injury because the stabilizing muscles that go along with the bicep are weak.

At each workout, always involve pushing and pulling exercises. For example if you do bench presses, also do seated rows to work the opposing muscles.

As much as you can, use more muscles rather than less. For example, rather than just standing doing dumbbell presses, put the weights on the ground and then lift them all the way back overhead with each repetition.

Use free weights more than machines. By avoiding machines, you work more stabilizing muscles, getting a better workout in less time. Most weight machines are useless. Use free weights whenever possible.

Always vary your workouts. Even if you are working the same muscles from workout to workout, don't do the same workout two days in a row. Find some way to vary it. For example, you can do the same workout but in reverse order. Also vary the number of repetitions and the amount of weight for each workout. For instance, on Monday you do squats for ten to twelve reps, but on Wednesday you do squats with heavier weight for one to five reps.

Change your exercises every month, and change your workouts with the seasons. So in winter you might like to cross-country or downhill ski, and in summer you might row. Vary it for the benefit of your mind and body.

Be off balance. Standing on a Bosu ball or a wobble board activates more muscles when performing an exercise. Instead of doing a standing press on the floor, you could stand on a wobble board to perform it. This will activate more muscles in the spine.

Chart your progress. Keep a workout journal so that you can challenge yourself to improve. It's also a good way to motivate yourself. By looking back you can see how you've improved.

Stretching

> But I will not go with you, because you are a *stiff-necked* people and I might destroy you on the way.
> —Exodus 33:3, emphasis mine

I realize God is using the term *stiff-necked* to indicate stubbornness, but you need to stretch every day if you want to be healthy. Perhaps God is trying to tell us to be spiritually and physically pliable (willing to change). He could have just said, "You are a stubborn people," but He didn't; I think God is sharing a practical truth. Muscles that are not flexible tear and rip much more easily when tested suddenly.

In fact, you should stretch twice each day. You need to stretch within a few minutes of waking up. Watch a cat or dog wake up, and you will see it stretch. Babies and young children automatically know how to stretch also. As we get older, this instinctive habit seems to diminish unless we make a conscious decision to stretch.

There are two kinds of stretching we will discuss: dynamic and static.

Dynamic Stretching

Dynamic stretching involves moving your joints to facilitate stretching. Dynamic stretches should be performed after you get out of bed. They involve repetition of movement.

The first stretch you should do is to arch backward, pause for one second, and then stretch forward, trying to touch your toes. Go slowly and controlled at first, and gradually speed up as it gets easier for you. As you arch backward, breathe in. As you bend forward, exhale. Perform the first five stretches twenty times each way. There is no holding this stretch. These types of stretches are designed to warm up joints, muscles, tendons, and ligaments.

Next, reach your hands over your head and bend to your side. Start nice and easy at first, gradually getting faster and farther with each stretch. Don't be surprised if body parts complain. If these are new to you, you probably will have some slight soreness at first. Be sure to drink a glass of water before you start; this will help.

The third stretch is the same as the previous one except your hands should be down and to your sides. Reach down the side of your leg as far as you can.

The fourth stretch requires that you interlace your fingers

and then hold your hands under your chin with your elbows straight out to the sides. Once more, stretch side to side.

For stretch number five put your hands on the sides of your head with your elbows out to the side. Tip your head and then your body side to side. Remember to do this twenty times each way.

The last warm-up stretch is to be performed twenty-five times each way. Cross your arms in front of you while standing with your feet shoulder width apart. Turn your head as far as you can to the right, and then twist your body. Go as far as you can then turn your head to the left and twist your body to the left. Don't twist your knees! Keep your head level.

There are other forms of dynamic stretches that you can do for your arms and legs. The principles are the same: move your joints through a full range of motion, and do an equal number for each motion.

Static Stretching

Static stretches are to be performed for thirty seconds to sixty seconds. These are the stretches where you assume a stretch and then hold it. There is little or no motion during a static stretch, hence the name. These types of stretches are best performed at the end of a workout when you are already warmed up. These stretches can be performed for every area of the body, but at the very least they should be performed for the major muscles.

Stretch your spine by flexing forward while sitting with your feet in front of you. Flip over onto your stomach and stretch back by using your arms to arch your back. Lie on your back and reach up with your hands, pointing your toes to make yourself as tall as you can. Twist your spine each way and hold. Stand with your feet on a stair and let you heals sink down to stretch your calf muscles. Pull your heel toward your buttock to stretch the front of your thigh. Stand up tall, and stretch your arms out and back so that you look like a "t."

Perform these stretches every day until the tight areas are not sore to stretch. To maintain your flexibility, remember to continue performing these at least once a week.

You should stretch to the point where you feel the muscles are tight and just a *little* uncomfortable. Don't push the stretch too much, or you could hurt yourself.

Yoga, tai chi and Pilates offer a good variety of stretching regimes, if you would like to be in a group setting.

Postural

Chiropractic doctors are not the only ones to understand that faulty or abnormal posture leads to poor health, but they have been correcting it the longest and understand it best. Many medical doctors and researchers are also promoting good posture for good health. It is important to correct abnormal posture or maintain normal posture because poor posture leads to tight muscles, abnormal joint wear and tear, increased stress on internal organs and nerves, and decreased energy and vitality.

Postural muscles are slow twitch muscles, so they need to be exercised differently from the fast twitch muscles that are used during strengthening exercises. Many rehabilitation programs now stress the importance of core stabilizing, with core being defined as the lower spine and abdomen. Unfortunately, many of these programs don't correct or align the spine before strengthening it, so the spine becomes strengthened in an abnormal (subluxated) position.

Pettibon rehabilitation procedures correct the spine alignment and the posture at the same time. These postural exercises should not be performed without proper Pettibon chiropractic care.

The most important postural exercises are performed using the Pettibon Body Weighting System ™ and are determined by a Pettibon doctor. These exercises are specific to the individual. It takes a minimum of ninety days to make a lasting change. The weights should be worn twice per day for twenty minutes at a time for best results. Once the correction is obtained, wearing the weights for twenty minutes once per week will maintain the muscle strength and endurance. Depending on the person's particular spine and posture abnormalities, he or she will need a combination of head, shoulder, and hip weights. In order to change the postural muscles, a person only has to wear the weights he or she needs. Wearing the weights on a Wobble Chair™ is beneficial, but a person can also walk around with the weights on.

A simple and effective postural exercise that anyone can perform almost anywhere is to simply stand up against a wall. The heels, buttocks, upper back, and head should all touch the wall while looking straight ahead. Hold the position for thirty to sixty seconds. Performing this daily will help improve posture, but it won't improve segmental spinal alignment.

Other Reasons to Exercise[38]

There are many other reasons to exercise, many of which are self-explanatory: exercise prevents diabetes, eliminates internal fat, prevents stroke, prevents heart disease, strengthens bones, prevents depression, improves blood pressure, improves flexibility, reduces arthritis pain, and improves balance. Plus, sitting shortens your life.

Exercise also helps with cancer reduction and new brain cell formation, and exercise honors God.

Cancer Reduction

Multiple studies show that even light to moderate exercise (thirty minutes of brisk walking five days per week) can decrease cancer risk significantly. The results were for colon, breast, pancreatic, endometrial, skin, and esophageal cancers.

New Brain Cell Formation

Exercise helps the body form new connections between brain cells, which also helps prevent dementia (Alzheimer's).

Honour God

One of the most frustrating things for me to hear about (and probably God also) is people who are unhealthy or sick and praying for healing who don't want to work at it. God can miraculously heal people from all kinds of illness. However, more often I think He wants us to learn how to take care of ourselves and avoid the need for major intervention. I don't think God will bless people when they just sit back in their easy chairs smoking cigarettes, drinking Cokes, eating bags of Doritos, and watching television. Instead, we should pray that God will free us from the bondage (smoking, junk food, etc.), and then we should do our utmost to avoid those things. When we are willing to make the effort to improve, God will bless us with better health.

The most important thing to remember about exercise is that you should *enjoy it*. Having fun will ensure that you continue. Also, exercise is a lifestyle, not some short-term nuisance to get you ready for bathing-suit season. If you want a long, active, and healthy life, don't ever stop exercising.

Exercise is necessary to stimulate changes in your body, but it's during rest that the improvements take place. In the next chapter, you will learn how to optimize rest and how to sleep so that you wake up feeling great and full of energy.

6 Sleep

… for He grants sleep to those He loves.
—Psalm 127:2

Does this chapter's epigraph mean that anyone who doesn't sleep well is not loved by God? I don't think so; God loves us all.

Sleep is interesting. It's something we do every day for approximately one third of our day, yet most of the time we don't think about how to do it correctly. Sleep is obviously important; otherwise, we wouldn't do it daily. It's during sleep that our bodies do most of the healing they require.

As I write this it is half past five in the morning, and I am a bit tired, but I have found that I perform the best on seven and a half hours of sleep. Soon I will fully awaken and forget about how comfortable my bed is. I enjoy the early morning hours. It's quiet and peaceful. I have also found that it's easier to commune with God.

Sleep is not as easy as it sounds for many people. In fact, it has become such a troublesome area of life and there are now so many sleep disorders that there are now "sleep experts," sleep clinics, and sleeping pills. According to Statistics Canada, one in seven (14 percent) Canadians over the age of fifteen has a sleep disorder. How is it that something that comes so naturally to us can become so troublesome?

In my practice, the number one reason why a parent would bring a baby to me is sleep related. Usually, the baby is waking up multiple times per night, making it hard for the parents (Mom mostly) to sleep. This lack of sleep leads to fatigue and, if it goes on too long, exhaustion.

Without proper sleep the immune system doesn't perform as well, so a person is more susceptible to infections. Most tired people are not cheerful and are less energetic, which means they are less productive. Lack of sleep can be dangerous when driving, and fatigue usually leads to overeating, which can cause diabetes and obesity.

Recently the head of a multi-city social support organization came to see me because of her poor sleep. Lucy* (age fifty-one) told me that for about five years she had been taking melatonin to try to sleep better, but it wasn't helping. The problem, she felt, was due to spinal discomfort. She was waking up five to six times per night. She was so low on energy that she wasn't able to get to work by half past eight in the morning. She went to the board of directors and asked them if she could start her work later in the day. This young regional director was so fatigued that she couldn't even get to work by half past eight! Even when she did make it to work, she reported that by midafternoon she was "out of it." In fact, her brain function was so impaired that she showed up an hour late for her initial appointment, even though she had it written down on an appointment card. She was only productive for four hours per day but was getting paid for eight. That's a lot of wasted time and money.

In order to get proper sleep, we need the right environment.

1. Lie down in a dark room: get thicker blinds or curtains for the summer months.
2. Make the space quiet: no television, no radio, no screaming kids, and no barking dogs.
3. Make sure you have a good bed: Most beds today are only good for ten years. Make sure your mattress is firm

---

* This is not her real name.

but has a pillow top. If you have a "no-flip" mattress, flip it every month and buy yourself a mattress topper for the other side. It will last you longer. Make sure you have a center support leg for the box spring to prevent sagging.

4. Go to bed with an empty bladder: do *not* drink caffeine in the evening, and be sure to drink enough water during the day.
5. Go to bed with an empty stomach: do *not* eat within one hour of bedtime.
6. Go to bed at a proper bedtime, which is around ten at night: Your quality of sleep will be better if you go to bed before midnight. Keep a regular bedtime all week, and don't blow it on the weekends. This is a hard one for shift workers.
7. Don't smoke.
8. Exercise: don't exercise within two hours of bedtime, but do exercise during the day, as you will sleep better.
9. Avoid drugs: avoid all kinds, because many prescription drugs disturb sleep.
10. Calm your mind: Avoid watching scary programs or reading frightening books. What goes into the mind the hour before we sleep significantly affects the brain and is remembered more easily. So *pray* before you go to bed and *read the Bible* to your kids and to yourself (the most important item on this list!).

What Is the Best Position for Sleep?

For babies and infants, side sleeping is best. Be sure to support them with cushions so they don't roll onto their stomachs. At around two years of age, children should start to sleep more on their backs. Ultimately the goal should be to sleep on your back. This is the most supportive position for the body with the least amount of twisting to the spine. Your pillow should be small and supportive to the neck without pushing your head forward.

Many people find they snore if the sleep on their backs. It is not normal to snore; it is, however, very common. If you snore, get a new pillow, improve your diet, get more exercise, and see a chiropractor. The wrong type of pillow can change the alignment of the neck, thereby changing the airway and leading to snoring. Food allergies or sensitivities could also be causing you to have sinus congestion, which leads to snoring. Being overweight is a common risk factor in snoring, so exercise more and eat better if you are overweight. Finally, vertebral subluxations can affect the function of the throat muscles, leading to snoring.

Snoring could also be due to swelling in the throat, such as swollen tonsils or adenoids. If they are swollen, don't get them removed; try to figure out why they are swollen.

Sleep should be a blessing. If it is not, you should get some help before it becomes hard to reestablish a normal sleep pattern. A special note to all you late night junkies, students, or people who like to cram as much as they can in a day: get a good night's rest, and you will enjoy the following day more. In nine years of college and university, I didn't drink coffee to stay up late studying. Even if I felt unprepared, I would get to bed on time and get up early to study more before the test. With a well-rested brain I was able to perform well on tests. Not to brag, but I graduated near the top of my class without depending on caffeine. In fact, I still don't drink more than one or two cups of coffee per month. Research confirms that we perform better when we get a good night's sleep.

Before getting chiropractic adjustments, I needed nine hours of sleep or I'd be a grouch. I had to sleep more because my body was not healthy. Now that I am healthy, I only sleep seven and a half hours and feel great. Remember, a healthy body functions as it should, so less sleep is needed.

I think the biggest key to good sleep can be found in Proverbs 3:21–24. "My son, preserve sound judgment and discernment, Do not let them out of your sight; They will be life for you, an ornament to grace your neck. Then you will go on your way in safety and your foot will not stumble; When you lie down, you will not be afraid; When you lie down, your sleep will be sweet." Psalm 4:8 also says, "I will lie down and sleep in peace, for you alone O LORD, make me dwell in safety."

Sleep also gives us a chance to forget our worries and troubles. It is almost as if we die to ourselves every night and are reborn every morning. We get to start over, so to speak, each day. Apparently people are sleeping less and less as we work increasingly more. Guard your sleep. On average, people are sleeping about one hour less today than we were a generation ago. If we don't sleep enough, we become mentally and physically impaired. Missing one hour of sleep impairs us to the same degree as one alcoholic drink does.

Another point to consider with sleep is the observance of the Sabbath, which is the one day we set aside for God, when we rest and enjoy a time of refreshing. It is the fourth commandment, not a suggestion. Whether you feel like you need it or not a day of rest and time with God is vital to good health. Some ideas for the Sabbath include spending time with your family, taking a nice walk, playing outside, engaging in a family game, or practicing devotions. Don't let legalism creep in though; as Jesus said, "I am the Lord of the Sabbath." Pray and seek God's will for the Sabbath.

Having the peace of God will allow you to sleep well. If you seek godly wisdom and live your life accordingly, you will go to bed with a clear conscience and sleep easier. This is a promise from God! Believe it.

In the next chapter you will discover that the greatest danger to your health might very well be right under your nose.

7

Air

Then the Lord God formed a man from the dust of the ground and breathed into his nostrils the breath of life, and the man became a living being.
-Genesis 2:7

All Scripture is God-breathed and is useful for teaching, rebuking, correcting and training in righteousness, [17] so that the servant of God[a] may be thoroughly equipped for every good work.
-2 Timothy 3:16-17

Obviously we need air to be healthy, but what most people don't know is that our homes are usually the worst places for air quality. Many people add "air fresheners" to their homes so that they will smell better, but these are usually made of toxic chemicals. Instead of adding toxic chemicals, clean the air in your home. The best way to clean the air is to vent the old stale air and bring fresh air in. This can be accomplished by opening windows and/or through the use of air exchangers through your furnace. Be sure to change or clean your furnace filter on a monthly basis to eliminate airborne particles.

If you live in an apartment or don't have a system in the house to draw fresh air in and filter it, you should purchase one or more free-standing air filters. The main feature to look for is the HEPA designation.

If you want your home to smell better, use natural essential oils. One of my favorites is grapefruit. It smells fresh, and most people don't have any allergies or sensitivities to it. There are many others available at health food stores and online. Find essential oils you like instead of the commercial toxic air sprays. Especially avoid the sprays that kill "germs"; if the chemicals are killing living organisms, they are also *toxic to us*.

If your home has a bad odor, you need to find out why. Common causes of foul odor in homes are mold, mice, pets, carpets, off gases from furniture and electronics, dirty laundry, and banana peels behind the couch. Find out if you can eliminate the source of the foul odor before you try to mask it with something else.

If you want to be healthy, you have to get outside every day and breathe in some fresh air. Even better, go for a walk outside. If you can't or don't want to walk for thirty minutes per day, at least go outside and take ten deep breaths.

Healthy Breathing

Many people don't breathe properly, which impairs their ability to get good oxygen saturation into their blood. Proper breathing is from the diaphragm and through the nose. Mouth breathing in children leads to a higher likelihood of dental problems. Table 1 outlines the many signs and symptoms of improper mouth and/or chest breathing. As you breathe in, your stomach should expand and then go back down when you exhale. Whenever you feel stressed, stop and take five to ten deep breaths. Breathe as deep as you can, and hold it in for a while. It is important that you don't breathe too quickly. Make sure that you aren't breathing with your upper chest because that will cause more tension. If you notice you are sucking your stomach in when you take a deep breath, you are chest breathing. Improper breathing can lead to increased stress to other areas of your body. Proper diaphragm breathing, however, will relieve stress.

Without proper diaphragm breathing, air doesn't get down to the lower recesses of the lungs. This increases your likelihood of a lung infection. Don't be surprised if you get some mucus coming up or feel like you have a cold when you improve your breathing. This is just your body getting rid of the buildup.

Table 1: Signs and Symptoms of Abnormal Breathing[39]

Weakness	Fatigue	Sleep disturbances	Blurred vision	Anxiety
Depression	Phobias	Feeling disconnected	Lightheaded	Dizziness
Disorientation	Seizures	Impaired thinking	Headaches	Palpitations
Chest pain	Tingling in the extremities	Difficulty breathing	Panic attacks	Sighing
Yawning	Dry mouth	Bloating	Belching	Flatulence
Cramping	Muscles spasms	Chest wall pain	Sleep apnea	Excessive plaque on front teeth
Sinus congestion	Plugged nose	Snoring	Upper shoulder and neck pain	High blood pressure

Nose breathing and using your diaphragm can help these types of issues to be resolved. Only about 10 percent of the population is breathing correctly, so take this seriously. If you improve your breathing you will live longer, because the diaphragm also helps to move blood up the heart. It acts like a second heart, moving blood from the feet to the heart. The better you breathe the less stress on your heart.

You will most likely need someone to help you retrain and monitor you. It takes twenty-one days to create a habit (if you use visualization and practice daily), so stick with it. Take

Dr. Davis E. Lindsay

a minute right now and check your breathing. Take a deep breath and see if your stomach moves, not your upper chest.

No amount of air will take away the mental hurts that build up inside. In the next chapter we will explore how to get your mind healthy. Learn how to get rid of the baggage that is dragging you down.

Mental Attitude

He who pursues righteousness and love finds life, prosperity and honor.

—Proverbs 21:21

He who is kind to the poor lends to the Lord, and He will reward him for what he has done.

—Proverbs 20:17

A cheerful heart is good medicine, but a crushed spirit dries up the bones.

—Proverbs 17:22

The book of Proverbs is full of great advice. I don't think it's a coincidence that there are thirty-one chapters, one for each day of the month. Some people are in the habit of reading a chapter every day, month after month. Personally, I read from Proverbs daily. Rather than read an entire chapter each day, I read a few verses so that I can remember them better. I read through the entire book twice a year.

Our attitudes and mental health are critical to our overall health. After all, we are body-mind-spirit, as discussed earlier. We can't disconnect our bodies from our minds or spirits, and we can't disconnect our minds from our bodies. Our mental health affects our physical health. We have such limited understanding that it's easier to break things down into parts to learn, but our body-mind-spirit operate simultaneously.

How much of all there is to know in the universe do you

think you know? I mean really know and understand fully. Do you think you know 10 percent? How about 1 percent? Do you think it's actually more like 0.0000000001 percent? I would say, for me, it's probably the last number. I know very little. Then there are all the things I know exist, but I don't really understand how they work. For example, I know that astronauts get launched out to the International Space Station, but I don't know what they do there, how far it is, what the training entails, or what rocket science they need to know. I know my car runs when I turn the key, but I don't know all the parts or how to put them together. I know there is food in the grocery store, but I don't know who picked the fruit or where the farm is. I could think of about twice as many things I don't know compared with what I do know.

Mostly, though, we don't know what we don't know. Over 99 percent of what God knows, I don't know even exists! We are all in the same boat. We know next to nothing. Yet we often act as if we know it all. Think of the city where you live; you probably can't name every street, but God can. He can actually tell you what is on every square millimeter of His planet, His solar systems, and His universe. He knows every person who ever was and is and will be. He knows *you*. He created you. He loves you! He has "plans to prosper you and not harm you."

Humility

We need to let go of our pride, because it will cause us grief. Remember that you know very little and that God gave you what you do know. Proverbs says, "Pride goes before destruction, a haughty spirit before a fall" (16:18). Earlier in the book, we read, "Do not be wise in your own eyes, fear the Lord and shun evil. This will bring health to your body and nourishment to your bones" (Proverbs 3:7–8). This is a promise from God to you. Humility will make you healthier.

Probably one of the best accounts of how pride leads to mental illness is found in Daniel 4. King Nebuchadnezzar is warned in a dream to protect himself from pride. Twelve months after his dream Nebuchadnezzar brags about how great Babylon is. He claims it is his "mighty power and for the glory of [his] majesty. The words were still on his lips when a voice came from Heaven." The king is driven from his people to live with wild animals, eating grass and living in the wilderness by himself. For seven years he doesn't cut his hair or nails. He roams around insane (out of touch with reality).

After seven years Nebuchadnezzar's "sanity is restored and his honor and splendor are returned to him." Daniel goes on to explain that Nebuchadnezzar "raised his eyes to heaven and honored and glorified the King of Heaven, because everything He does is right and all His ways are just. And those who walk in pride He is able to humble." That's a hard way to learn a lesson, but God "restored his throne and he became even greater than before."

Common Insanity

When we are out of touch with reality or truth, we become insane. When a majority of the population becomes out of touch with the truth, I call that "common insanity". More recently it has been said that we live in a "post truth" era, where people will ignore the truth or not seek truth if something doesn't suit their beliefs. For example, at one time most people thought that the earth was flat. Those who thought so were suffering from common insanity. Those who sought the truth were labeled insane by those who were insane. Ironic, isn't it?

Today most people believe that drugs will make them well. I used to believe this also, but I discovered that it is not true; it is common insanity. There are drugs that can save a life, but taken for longer periods does not restore health. Yet those of us (and there are many) who tell the truth are often ridiculed. It doesn't bother me because I seek my praise from God, not from people. I seek to do what is right in God's eyes. I don't always succeed. When I make mistakes, I turn back to God and ask for forgiveness and try to do better.

It is so easy to allow the mistakes and hurts of our pasts to haunt us. We must let them go. The only way we can really do that is to ask God to take them. Jesus died to take away our transgressions, sins, debts, trespasses, and mistakes. Only when we are in a healthy relationship with Jesus can we be fully forgiven and be fully alive and well. There is no other substitute.

The Stress Reaction

Under stress our body creates stress hormones. As stress hormones increase our ability to regulate blood sugars decreases, our bodies become more resistant to insulin, our body produces fewer insulin receptors on our cells, our blood pressure goes up, our blood sugar levels increase, blood clotting factors increase, muscle and connective tissue breakdown occurs. We become depressed, our immune system becomes impaired, our resistance to diseases goes down, our cholesterol levels increase, our frontal lobe brain function decreases (making it harder to learn or remember), our eyes dilate, we become over stimulated making it harder to sleep, serotonin levels decrease, our sensitivity to pain increases, growth hormone and testosterone levels decrease and we crave fats and sugars.

These types of changes are helpful during a short period of stress such as when some encounters a bear. After the bear leaves we calm down and these levels should go back to normal. The problem is that most people are now chronically stressed. We are in this fight or flight mode basically every day, all day and even while we sleep. Too much stress for too long leads to burn out, diabetes, heart disease, obesity, impotence, sleep problems, dementia, depression, immune problems, blood clotting disorders and high blood pressure.

Gratitude

Negative thinking, such as complaining, increases our stress-hormone levels, which leads to many negative health effects, but gratitude decreases our stress hormones. I used to have a hard time feeling grateful for the things in my life. Instead I found it easier to dwell on what I didn't have. I had created a habit of envy. Like any bad habit, it just sort of happens slowly over time. And before you know it, it becomes automatic. I had hard-wired negativity into my brain just as one hard-wires how to ride a bike—by constantly working at it.

How God opened my eyes to my negativity was through a poor little woman living in a slum in India. I saw a picture of her in a magazine in which she was sitting on a pile of garbage, eating someone else's discarded food. She had a great big grin on her face, the kind you see on people after they win the lottery. But she didn't win the lottery; she lived in a garbage dump eating other people's garbage. She was thankful for what she had. I had a million times more than her, and here I was unsatisfied and wanting more. I was a fool! That's when I decided to change.

I started writing down the things I was grateful for. At first I only had one or two things, but gradually it grew. Every morning I would write in my journal the blessings I had received from God the day before. Now I can think of many things I am grateful for, but I usually limit myself to just ten. If you can't think of anything to be grateful for, then be grateful that you don't live in a garbage dump. Brain researchers tell us it takes a minimum of about twenty-one days to create a habit. So commit to do this for twenty-one days. Try it, and before you know it you will start being more grateful, less stressed and healthier.

Having done this for many years now, it is easy to see the good in almost every situation because I have trained myself to see it. But it wasn't always easy. As a young man I was often depressed and gloomy. I still have my moments, but we should be sad about things that are sad. Emotions are what make us human, but we shouldn't be constantly stressed.

Crying Is Good

What's better for you, crying or laughing? They both are. Crying is a reflex that our bodies use to release negative stress. One of the worst things a parent can do to a child is to tell him or her not to cry when sad or hurt. Please don't do that to your kids. When a person finishes crying, he or she releases the stress. If a person is told not to cry, the stress stays indefinitely ... unless he or she deals with it at some later date. Plus, scolding kids for crying also teaches them (especially boys) that it is best to bottle up emotions and pretend everything is fine.

Crying is a reflex similar to other reflexes. Our unconscious brain controls it to help our bodies become healthier. Coughing and sneezing allow our bodies to get rid of harmful things. Is it good to keep in a sneeze? No, not at all! What happens if we don't allow our bodies to cough? We allow an infection or debris to stay trapped in our lungs, which leads to more illness. So instead of a mild chest infection, it becomes deadly pneumonia. That's why you should never use cough syrup, and that's why a person should always cry when needed. Get it out!

Laughter Really Is the Best Medicine

Laughter is good medicine. It has no side effects. Well, maybe your sides do get affected if you laugh a lot (sore muscles). Seriously, laughter will do more good for a person's health than any drug could. *Laughter is the only medicine we should ever take*, and we should get some every day and in large doses. So make it a habit to laugh a lot daily.

Following are some verses about laughter. Genesis 21:6 says, "Sarah said, 'God has brought me *laughter*, and everyone who hears about this will laugh with me'" (emphasis mine). Job 5:22 says, "You will *laugh* at destruction and famine and need not fear the beasts of the earth" (emphasis mine). Psalm 2:4 "The One enthroned in heaven *laughs* …" (emphasis mine). Psalm 126:2 says, "Our mouths were filled with *laughter*, our tongues with songs of joy" (emphasis mine). Ecclesiastes 3:4 says there is "a time to weep and a time to *laugh*" (emphasis mine). There are others, but you get the point: God invented laughter for our benefit, and He laughs too.

> Knock, knock. Who's there? Olive. Olive who? Olive you!

> Even corny jokes can bring a smile to your face.

> Two hats were hanging on a hat rack in the hallway. One hat said to the other: "You stay here; I'll go on a head."

> I wondered why the baseball kept getting bigger. Then it hit me.

Love

Did you know that without love you would die? "God is Love" (1 John 4:8). Therefore, without love we would have no God, and without God, no love. When God is gone, life is gone. Studies have shown that without love people have shorter life expectancies, more illness, more likelihood of suicide, and more depression, and babies who are deprived love fail to thrive.

We all need to love and be loved. Married people live longer than unmarried. Even if you only love a pet, it will improve your mental, physical, and spiritual health. You have probably heard of or have known someone who had been married for many years and then died soon after his or her spouse died. When losing the love of one's life, one often loses the desire to live.

Sometimes in our desire for love we turn to relationships that are not healthy simply because someone seems to care for us. Before you enter into a marriage, be sure you already have a healthy relationship with God. Otherwise you could end up "settling" for someone who fills the void right now.

There is some confusion as to what love really means. The world's version of love is not God's description. The world says, "If you love me, I will love you a little. Or if you do nice things for me, I will love you. Or as long as you look pretty ... Or ..." In contrast, 1 Corinthians 13 describes God's love for us in a way that we are to pass on to others: "Love is patient, love is kind. Love does not envy, it does not boast, it is not proud. Love is not rude, it is not self-seeking, it is not easily angered, it keeps no record of wrongs. Love does not delight in evil but rejoices with the truth. Love always protects, always trusts, always hopes, always perseveres. Love never fails ... And now these three remain: faith, hope and love, but the greatest of these is love" (4–8, 13).

We can't truly love on our own unless we know God and have His love in us. I believe that babies are full of godly love because they come from heaven. But unless they are constantly refilled with this love, they become depleted. By nature, we all fall short and are sinful from birth unless we call on God to fill us with His Spirit of love.

Love is not a noun but a verb, an action word. In order to love we have to be "doing" love. Sometimes we may not actually love someone, but if we act as if we do then we may start to love. God proved His love for us when He sent His Son to die for us while we were still sinners. We need to do the same. Love others even when they don't love you. Give even if you don't receive.

"The love you give is the love you keep," says B. J. Palmer, a chiropractic doctor.

Now, that doesn't mean you should be in abusive relationships. You can love someone and not be near the person. Love your ex-spouse, but you don't have to talk to him or her every day. Love the person who fired you from your job. Love the person begging for help, whom you drive by every day. Love the politicians you didn't vote for. Love the police officer who gave you a ticket for breaking the law. Love the person you are married to even though he or she isn't perfect. Meet your spouse's needs, and watch him or her grow more in love with you. Husbands, love your wives; wives, respect your husbands. Don't let divorce be an option, except for those situations that involve continual infidelity, abuse or danger to yourself or children. Love and live; love and be healthy.

David had to love Saul even though Saul was hunting him day and night. Talk about an abusive relationship. Spears were thrown at him while he was eating dinner! David trusted God even when he could have killed Saul himself. David loved Saul even when there was no reason to.

Contentment

Being greedy and dissatisfied breeds discontent and mental stress. There are times when God will make us feel uneasy with our current situation to stir us to change. That's a good thing, but being jealous of others is not good. As the Bible says, "A heart at peace gives life to the body, but envy rots the bones" (Proverbs 14:30).

We must be careful not to be jealous or envious. Being content or at peace gives us life, but not being content makes us sick. Envy literally causes us to become sick. Research has shown that having these kinds of negative emotions causes cancer, heart disease, high blood pressure, diabetes, colds, infections, depression, premature gray hair, and other issues. That's the way it is with God. Follow His ways and be blessed; follow your own and be cursed. Be at peace and be well.

Strive to improve for God's sake—not to get more material things, but to get more spiritual blessings. Jesus said, "Seek first His kingdom and His righteousness and all these things will be

Dr. Davis E. Lindsay

given to you as well" (Matthew 6:33). When we put God first, everything else in our lives will line up and improve.

It's Better to Give Than Receive

Giving back to your community is a great way to improve your mental health. Volunteering is a great way to be connected to others, to see needs, and to share God's love with the world. As if those weren't enough good reasons to help out, God hard-wired our brains to need to give. In other words, if we aren't volunteering, we are slowing becoming depleted. We need to refill our "giving tanks" weekly. It's impossible to be healthy by only taking; we have to give. And when we give, we are also blessed by it.

Think of giving like showering: it helps get rid of the dirt that builds up on us, including the dirt of ungratefulness, feeling sorry for ourselves, pride, selfishness, and greed. If we don't wash it off weekly, it starts to build up a stinky crust that repels others and eventually ourselves.

You can volunteer at your church, a food bank, as a coach, at a school, and so on—the list is endless. Pray and ask God to show you where He wants you to be; I guarantee you will be glad you did. As the Bible says, "He who oppresses the poor shows contempt for their Maker, but whoever is kind to the needy honors God" (Proverbs 14:31).

Having Fun

Rejoice in the Lord always; again I will say, rejoice!
—Philippians 4:4

Joy is a command in Philippians 4:4. We are to rejoice, meaning we are to be filled with joy. Focus on the good things in your life and be happy, no matter what is going on in your life. Worry about nothing; pray about everything.

"Having Fun" is the last section in this chapter because this

90

was the last area of my attitude that I needed to get right. I grew up and one day realized I wasn't having fun. I was too worried about my finances, my family, the planet, etc. My sense of humor was lukewarm at best, and I was too serious. I needed to act like a kid and enjoy life again. I bet you could have more fun too.

How old would you be if you didn't know how old you are? Too many of us are acting like we are old farts even when we are young. Don't grow up, stop taking yourself too seriously, and have fun. Being too serious will age you, and you will miss out on life's joys.

Play with Legos; go bungee jumping; jump on a trampoline; play a harmonica or any instrument you can; play a silly game, such as hide and go seek (in the dark with flashlights); throw a ball for a dog, or chase a little kid around. Whatever is fun for you, just do it.

To learn how to get your physical body clean and avoid toxic chemicals in the process, turn to the next chapter.

Hygiene

You shall also make a basin of bronze, with its stand of bronze, for *washing*. You shall put it between the tent of meeting and the altar, and you shall put water in it.

—Exodus 30:18

When it comes to being clean, we need to be careful not to use dangerous (toxic) chemicals on our bodies. Basic soap and water will take care of most dirt on our bodies. Today it's hard to find "basic soap." We buy ours from a local soap maker who uses simple, natural, and healthy ingredients, such as olive oil, goat's milk, and rose petals. It smells nice and gets us clean. Most commercial soaps have toxic chemicals in them. The fragrance, artificial colors, and other chemicals are detrimental to our health.

When choosing your shampoo and conditioner, consider the ingredients; what we put on our bodies goes into our bodies. Our skin absorbs it, and then it enters our bloodstream. Putting something on our skin is analogous to eating it. So if you shouldn't eat it, don't put it on your skin. There are products now that are mostly made of plant or animal oils. For example, I have seen lip balm made of emu oil. But instead of buying some overpriced item, just get coconut oil to put on your skin or lips. It is edible and healthy and is much less costly.

The most important thing to remember about skin health is it comes from the *inside*. Consider the advertisements for dog food that we have discussed in previous chapters. How does food improve the look of a dog's coat or, for that matter, your hair? Well, the nutrients needed for healthy hair come from the food. If the food has the right nutrients, we will be healthy on the inside and out. If you want healthy skin, improve your diet. Save your money on all the creams, lotions, and potions, and buy healthy food. Get your essential omega-3 fats, and drink enough water. Dry skin is often telling you that you are dehydrated. If your lips are chapped, drink more water. Most skin lotions and conditioners contain alcohol, which dries out your skin or hair and thus causes the problem to continue.

Our skin is also a means for our bodies to eliminate toxins. If our kidneys, lungs, and bowels aren't able to eliminate fast enough, our skin will be utilized. One of the functions of sweating is to get rid of toxins. So sweat, daily. You can do that with saunas or hot tubs, but exercise is the best way to sweat. And yes, it is okay for ladies to sweat too. The more toxic a person is, the smellier he or she will be upon sweating. Putting a cup of Epsom salts in the bath is a good way to draw out toxins. Certain skin conditions are due to the body trying to eliminate toxins.

Certain neurologic disorders can lead to skin abnormalities also. Shingles and cold sores are the most common ones caused by a weakness in the body's ability to fight off the herpes virus. The herpes virus lives in the nerves but can only create problems when the immune system is not able to suppress it. The problem will usually come from some type of stress: physical, emotional, or chemical stress. The physical stress can be from subluxations that interfere with proper nerve function. Subluxations can interfere with kidney, bowel, or liver function, which impairs our ability to eliminate toxins in the typical way. The healthier our spines are, the healthier our skin will be.

The condition of our vascular systems will also affect our skin. With poor circulation, skin cells are not going to be healthy. The most common disorder in this regard is diabetes. Nerve endings die due to lack of circulation, and poor circulation leads to tissue death. Many people with diabetes lose their lower limbs. In 2007, according to the American Diabetes

Association, 71, 000 Americans had a limb amputated due to poor circulation.

Deodorant is another product to be cautious with. Many commercial deodorants and so-called "natural crystal" deodorants contain aluminum. It's usually on the label as potassium alum. The full chemical name is potassium aluminum sulphate. Aluminum has been shown to be toxic to people even in small doses; it has been linked to brain disorders, such as dementia or Alzheimer's, and it has a possible link to breast cancer.[40]

Even worse than a deodorant that masks the smell is antiperspirant, which actually stops your body from perspiring. We need to sweat to cool down and eliminate toxins, so don't put toxins on your skin to stop you from getting rid of toxins.

If you stop using deodorants and antiperspirants, you will notice that "pit" stains will not be on your shirts anymore. You will still sweat, but if you wash your armpits each day or after exercise with soap and water, you will probably not be stinky. If you still are, that means there are other toxins to be eliminated; you should do a cleansing fast (see chapter 3).

Can you be too clean? Yes, you can. Usually this stems from an irrational fear of germs ("germophobia"). There are far more healthy germs than harmful. When a person constantly washes, he or she gets rid of the good germs as well as the bad. Don't use alcohol-based hand sanitizers, as they damage the skin and kill the good germs too. Good old soap and water are all that is needed. And don't use the anti-bacterial soaps, as they contain antibiotics and other toxins.

We buy our soap from a local family who makes all their own soaps and sells them at our farmer's market. The list of ingredients is fairly simple: a plant oil, usually olive; an animal fat (usually cream); lye (sodium hydroxide); and some natural essential plant oil for smell (lavender, geranium, etc.). Or you can make your own soap. Lye can be made from hardwood ashes; after all, that's how it was done roughly five thousand years ago. The point is to avoid all the toxins that most major soap maker use.

It is also not necessary to wash your hair every day, as this will usually dry it out. Look at the list of ingredients in shampoos and conditioners; there are a lot of chemicals. If you sweat from exercise or work, go ahead and shower, but you don't have to use a cleaning product on your head; just water will do. Use shampoo and conditioner every second or third day instead.

Brush Your Teeth with Candy

Most commercial toothpastes are full of sweeteners. These sweeteners are usually artificially made in a lab. How does that make sense? Dentists tell us to avoid sweets, and then we are supposed to go clean our teeth with sweeteners. The reasoning is that artificial sweeteners don't cause damage to the teeth as sugars can. Maybe this is so, but now you have toxic chemicals in your mouth, which get absorbed into the bloodstream. Substances that go into the mouth or under the tongue get quickly absorbed, so don't think you are safe as long as you don't swallow. There are healthier options in most health food stores. Or if you want to make your own healthy toothpaste, all you need is a bit of baking soda and mint oil. Also you can dilute hydrogen peroxide and gargle with it. Just use a teaspoon of hydrogen peroxide in four ounces (125 milliliters) of water.

Even better yet, get yourself a toothbrush that doesn't require toothpaste. We have been using a Soladey toothbrush for over a year now and have noticed improved cleaning of our teeth and decreased use of toothpaste. It doesn't have any nasty fluoride or sugars, it's better for the environment (since we're not throwing away toothpaste bottles), and it's less expensive. (Go to soladey.com for more information.)

Mercury Fillings

Most people with chronic horrible illnesses have mouths full of mercury. Mercury fillings can leach into the bloodstream, creating a whole host of health problems, including cancer, Parkinson's, ALS, dementia, heart attacks, fibromyalgia, infections, and chronic fatigue.

According to the World Health Organization (WHO), mercury can cause serious health effects, even in small amounts and especially to developing babies, in utero. Mercury can have toxic effects on the nervous system, digestive system, immune system, lungs, kidneys, skin, and eyes. The WHO recommends the discontinuation of mercury use in dental fillings.[41] If you want to find a dentist who is more holistic and natural in your area, go to holisticdentist.org.

If you want to take your spiritual health to a new level, read the next chapter.

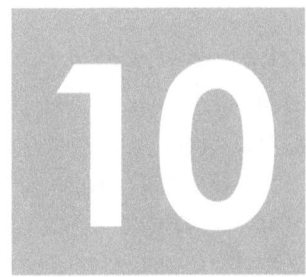

Spiritual Health

Jesus answered, "I am the way and the truth and the life. No one comes to the Father except through me..."

-John 14:6

Currently there are two prevailing ideas about the origin of life: creation or evolution. Both require a leap of faith. Evolution is a leap of faith whereby a person believes that by some astronomically small chance, our planet and all the others were formed. The Theory of Evolution assumes that we evolved from a primordial soup. Life started as a simple organism and just gradually evolved over millions of years. Statisticians have determined that it is so unlikely that the planets could have come into being by a random chance that it takes more faith to believe in this idea than it would to believe in creation. If Earth were moved closer or farther from the sun by even one thousand feet, it would not sustain life. When you study the movement of the stars and planets you quickly realize that there is a predictable pattern and order to the universe. The sign of a creator. Taking drugs hoping to get healthier is also a leap of faith. Some people take drugs instead of trusting their bodies to heal themselves.

On the other hand, believing in God requires a leap of faith to believe in a being who is all powerful, all knowing, and ever present. At first it's not much easier to believe in God; after all, where is He? Many people argue that believing in God is a weakness. But what if God does really exist; then what?

If God really does exist and is omnipotent, omniscient, and omnipresent, shouldn't we be able to sense Him? I believe we were all born with a longing to know that God is real and sense His presence. To believe in a God who created us for a specific purpose, loves us, and is watching out for us is a much more comforting and fulfilling worldview.

This is probably the easiest way I know of proving God's existence. Get yourself into a room by yourself with no noise to distract you. Close your eyes. Relax and breathe. Now focus on the colour black. Now imagine nothing. Imagine absolute blackness where nothing exists. There is no air or dust; there are no microorganisms or particles—just nothing. Okay? Now imagine a living cell. It's alive; inside are a multitude of tiny organelles keeping that cell alive. That cell needs nutrients, where did they come from? Now imagine planets, stars, moons, and a sun. How did they get there from nothing? It's *impossible* to create something from nothing. One of the Laws of Physics states that matter can't be created or destroyed. So how did the universe come to be? They had to be created.

Now try this, take a big box of Lego building blocks and dump it onto the floor. How long do you think it would take before anything was created? How about a simple Lego house? A Lego car? Anything? Try dumping out a box of Lego a billion times, there still would be just a random pile of blocks.

Every living cell, whether from a plant or animal is very complex and has an intelligent design to it and is interconnected to just about everything else on Earth. Even if there were billions of years to accomplish the task, you still can't create something from nothing. The evolution theory tries to convince us that given enough time, creation will happen. Many scientists are now coming to the realization that evolution couldn't have created the known universe. Unfortunately for them, they don't want to admit the existence of a Creator. The Bible contains over 300 prophecies (or predictions) about the life of Jesus Christ that were written hundreds of years before his birth and by multiple authors. In 1952 Peter Stoner used the science of probability and statistics to determine that for just 8 prophecies about Jesus to be fulfilled would be one chance in 10,000,000,000,000,000,000,000,000,000,000 (that's 28 zeros). Essentially it would have been impossible, but that is for just 8 prophecies. When you consider 48 prophecies the number becomes a one with 157 zeros after it. He says that if you were to make a ball of electrons (which are so small you can fit 2500 trillion in an inch) you would create a ball that extends "in all directions to the distance of six billion light-years 6×10^{28} times." That's only for 48 prophecies there are over 300. It's impossible to get all those right by chance. Mr. Stoner's work has been reviewed and verified by H. Hartzler P.h.D.[42]

When people don't know God, they try to fill the emptiness with other things: travel, relationships, hobbies, music, movies, games, sports, and religion. Following a set of rules doesn't mean that a person knows God. The Son of God was crucified by the religious rulers of His day. Don't confuse religion with spiritual health. Spiritual health is about a sense of belonging and purpose. It is about accepting that you are not perfect but accepting who you are: a unique and important creation, a child of God. Spiritual health is about receiving forgiveness through Jesus and trying to better yourself as a person by following the example set by Him; the only perfect person to ever live. Spiritual health is about love, joy, peace, contentment, forgiveness, gratitude, humility, selflessness, giving, caring, fellowship, and being in a relationship with God, the Creator.

When a person has a relationship with God, he or she doesn't have the same fears and anxieties about the future. Before I met God, I would often worry about death. It would become more real to me whenever someone I knew passed away. I would wonder, *is he or she going to heaven or hell? Do these places exist? Will I go to heaven?* All of these things led me to times of despair and depression. It wasn't until I met God that I was able to fully achieve peace in my life. I used to have high blood pressure, but now I don't. It's not that I wasn't eating well or exercising; the stress of uncertainty was affecting my physical and mental health.

Hearing God

There is an account of a little boy named Samuel in the Old Testament book, 1 Samuel. Samuel hears a voice whispering to him one night. At first he believes that it is the voice of his guardian, Eli. After hearing the voice several times and being told by his teacher that it must be the voice of God, Samuel responds to the voice by saying, "Speak, for your servant is listening" (1 Samuel 3:10 NIV). God then speaks to Samuel! The Creator of the universe speaks to His creation. I have heard God speak to me at times also, which is how I know He is real. I know that a lot of psychotic people have said that God told them to kill someone, so it is with great reservation that I share this. However, I have spoken to other perfectly sane people who have also heard the voice of God.

When God speaks to people, it is usually not a loud boom-ing voice but a quiet, inner voice. It's usually when we are alone and wanting to hear from Him that He whispers. I be-lieve that He speaks to all of us, but most of us miss it. Some people will call it "intuition" or a sense or feeling about some-thing. They will often say things like, "I don't know why, but I feel I should do _____." His voice is a lot like our own, but it's always loving, always caring, and always true.

The first time I heard God's voice, He saved my life. This was before I even believed that God existed. I was going through a particularly depressing time in my life. A young woman I wanted to be in a relationship with had rejected me. I was devastated. I was driving along a highway that runs next to a river, a stretch of road that has taken many lives when the weather is bad. The cold, deep, dark waters are unforgiving. I thought to myself, *I can just drive into the river, and all this pain and sadness will be over. Besides, I'm insignificant. If life is*

102

just going to hand me more pain and suffering as time passes, I might as well check out early. I didn't believe in eternity. I just figured death was the end. But then I heard a voice ask, "What about your parents? They will be devastated."

There it was; I heard it. It was a voice inside my mind not unlike the voice I hear when I am thinking or reading quietly. We all have that voice, but this was different. It sounded a lot like my inner voice, but it wasn't me. So I started thinking about how awful my death would be to my parents. They have always been loving, supportive, and good to me. I had seen the pain caused by suicide in other families, so I decided to just carry on with life.

That also got me to thinking about the source of that voice. Was I mentally ill? Or did God exist? I started thinking about it more and more. I asked questions; I wanted to know. If there were a God, this would change everything about my life. Well, God put a great friend into my life at that time. He already had a relationship with God, and he told me to challenge God to prove that He exists. He reasoned that if the Creator could speak the universe into being, He could speak to me. Look at Genesis 1, starting in verse 3: "And God said, 'let there be light,' and there was light." The words *God said* appear eight more times in chapter 1. After each time He spoke, something was created! God spoke the sun, the moon, the stars, the planets, and everything on them into being.

God spoke to me a second time. It was about a year after the first time. I took the challenge and asked God to prove Himself to me. About a week later, I was getting onto a very full bus as a lady was getting off the wrong way. Instead of going out the side door, she was coming right up to the front where I and several other people were getting on. I noticed her because it's awkward when people are trying to get on a cramped bus and someone is going against the flow. She passed by several people, and when she got up to me she stopped and looked me in the eyes with these incredible sky blue eyes. It felt like she was looking into my soul. Then she said it: "God told me to tell you that He loves you!" That was it. As fast as it happened, it was over, and she was gone off the bus. I went and sat down at the back of the bus, stunned. Was this just some religious wacko who does this to everyone? No. I had asked God for proof. This wasn't a coincidence. She didn't talk to anyone else; she singled me out.

I now knew God was real, by faith. I still didn't know Him very well. I thought I did, but I had a lot of learning to do. For example, I thought God was this big, mean ruler of the universe looking down at people and just waiting for them to screw up so He could punish them. I thought He was far off and aloof, someone you could never know. Boy, was I wrong. I didn't realize God wanted a relationship with me, not religion. He wants a relationship with you too.

When we are in tune with God, we can't help but feel alive. We don't have to feel the burdens of the world. Having a solid relationship takes time, but it gives us so much in return.

Another example of God speaking to people comes from the account of Moses in the book of Exodus. It is full of conversations between God and Moses. My favorite from these is Exodus 33:11, which says, "The LORD would speak to Moses face to face, as a man speaks with his friend." How amazing and beautiful! Speaking to God can be like speaking face to face with a friend. Then I read Hebrews 1:1–2, which says, "In the past *God spoke* to our forefathers through the prophets at many times and in various ways, but in these days He has spoken to us by His son, whom He appointed heir of all things and through whom He made the universe" (emphasis mine).

Make the time every day to speak to your friend, your God. Eventually, you will be able to converse with God just as Moses did. I was jealous. Why did Moses get to talk to God like that and not me? Well, like any relationship, it took time to develop before it became a beautiful friendship. If you are having a hard time hearing His voice, at least read His word; He speaks through that also. God also speaks through dreams and visions, so pay attention to them.

Promises You Can Count On

The Bible is full of God's promises to us. One of my favorites is "Never will I leave you, never will I forsake you" (Hebrews 13:5). When we choose to love and serve God, we can be sure that no matter what happens He will always be there for us: "'For I know the plans I have for you,' declares the Lord, 'plans to prosper you and not to harm you. Plans to give you hope and a future. Then you will call upon me and come and pray to me and I will listen to you. You will seek me and find me when you seek me with all your heart'" (Jeremiah 29:11–13).

God expects us to treat others the way we want to be treated. If we do, He promises rewards. For example, Isaiah 58:7–9 says, "Is it not to share your food with the hungry and to provide the poor wanderer with shelter—when you see the naked, to clothe him, and not to turn away from your own flesh and blood? Then your light will break forth like the dawn, and your healing will quickly appear; then your righteousness will go before you, and the glory of the Lord will be your rear guard. Then you will call and the Lord will answer; you will cry for help, and He will say: Here am I."

How can we expect God to do what we want if we don't do what He wants? After all, He knows better. God always wants to give us our best life. The world will offer us good, but God offers us His best. Don't choose second place; claim what God wants you to have. Proverbs 28:25 says, "He who trusts in the Lord will prosper." And 29:25 says, "Whoever trusts in the Lord is kept safe."

It can be hard to trust in God, but we must always remember that everything He does is because He loves us. We are His children and creation. In the popular Psalm 23, David illustrates a beautiful example of God's love: "The Lord is my shepherd ... He restores my soul."

Sheep are a funny animal. If they fall over, it is almost impossible for them to stand up again. If they end up on their backs, they frantically flail about and cry for help. If they can't get up, gas begins to collect in their stomachs. Eventually their stomachs get so full of air that their airways get cut off, which could lead to suffocation. This is referred to as the "cast down" position.

When the shepherd comes along, he or she speaks to the sheep to calm it, massages its legs to improve circulation, gently turns it over, lifts it on its feet again, and holds it so it can regain it balance. This is what God does for us. When we are down and out and flailing around because of our own mistakes (guilt, grudges, or grief), our loving shepherd reassures us with His grace, lifts us up, and holds us until we've regained our spiritual equilibrium.

If you are cast down for any reason, let God get you back on your feet again. He will restore your soul with confidence, joy, peace, and strength.[43]

If you want to know what joy is, observe a young child around three years old. A child that young isn't worried about the stock market or about his or her hair, clothes, or future. Young children are usually filled with a zest for life that bubbles over into everything they do.

Early on in the Old Testament God declares to all people who follow Him, "I am the LORD who heals you" (Exodus 15:26). I think it is important to remember that the first half of that verse says, "If you listen carefully to the voice of the LORD your God and what is right in his eyes, if you pay attention to His commands and keep all His decrees, I will not bring on you any of the diseases I brought on the Egyptians, for I am the LORD who heals you." If we live godly lives, we can expect blessings; if not, we will bring curses on ourselves.

Fear God?

Do not be wise in your own eyes; *fear the Lord* and shun evil. This will bring health to your body and nourishment to your bones.
—Proverbs 3:7–8, emphasis mine

> *The fear of the Lord*—that is wisdom, and to shun
> evil is understanding.
> —Job 28:28, emphasis mine

It seems a little odd to fear God. After all, He is our heavenly Father. God is love, so why fear Him? Lack of fearing God can lead to our destruction. Pharaoh wanted all the Hebrew boys killed, but "the midwives, however, *feared God* and did not do what the king of Egypt told them to do … So God was kind to the midwives" (Exodus 1:17, 20, emphasis mine).

Here is an example of a time when someone didn't fear God: "But Er, Judah's firstborn, was wicked in the Lord's sight; so the Lord put him to death" (Genesis 38:7). If Er had feared God, he wouldn't have done wicked things. I think what it boils down to is a single question: do you believe that God is *all seeing*? If you don't, you will do wrong and not worry about it. But if you believe that God sees all you do, you will try to avoid making mistakes or breaking His commandments.

In 2 Samuel 11 and 12, we read the account of David coveting Bathsheba (a married woman). David committed adultery with her and then sent her husband to the front lines of a battle to be killed: "the thing David had done displeased the Lord" (2 Samuel 11:27). God sent Nathan to give David a warning from God. Nathan then asked David, "Why did you *despise* the word of the Lord by doing what is evil in His eyes?" (emphasis mine). God punished David in several ways for his adultery and murder: "Therefore, the sword will never depart from your house, because you *despised* me and took the wife or Uriah the Hittite to be your own" (2 Samuel 12:9–10, emphasis mine). David confessed his sins to God, to which Nathan replied, "The Lord has taken away your sin. You are not going to die … the son born to you will die" (2 Samuel 12:13–14, emphasis mine). God forgave David, but the child born from adultery was taken back to heaven to be with God.

Now it might seem cruel for a child to die for the sins of the father, but God is always just and fair. Everything He does, He does out of love. The death of the child was a reminder to David, the king of a nation, to change his attitude. Otherwise an even worse fate would have befallen an entire nation. The child went directly to heaven and was probably spared a life of shame and agony. He would have been labeled the child of an adulterous act and would have been despised by many.

That's not the end of the story. David and Bathsheba conceived again, but this time they did so as a married couple. About this child, the Bible says, "The Lord loved him" (2 Samuel 12:24). He was named Solomon by his parents, but God named him Jedidiah, meaning *loved by the Lord*. This child was born to the same parents, as witnessed by the same God, but his were totally different circumstances. This shows the damage of sin and the power of repentance and forgiveness.

Another example comes from Jeremiah 32:39–41, which says, "I will give them singleness of heart and action, so that they will always fear me for their own good and good of their children after them. I will make an everlasting covenant with them: I will never stop doing good to them and I will inspire them *to fear me, so that they will never turn away from me*. I will rejoice in doing them good and will assuredly plant them in this land with all my heart and soul" (emphasis mine). You see, it is for our own good that we fear God; otherwise we will turn away from Him.

God goes on to say in chapter 33, "I will bring health and healing; I will heal my people and will let them enjoy abundant peace and security" (6). It is our choice whether to follow or not. God will not force us. Sometimes people think freedom away from God is better, but it is not.

If you have any sins between you and God, repent and be forgiven. Start now. Remember your mistakes, learn from them, but don't dwell on them. Accept the forgiveness that God offers through Jesus' death on the cross.

We should also fear God because He holds eternity in His hands. If we choose to ask for forgiveness we will spend eternity in paradise with God, but if we reject His forgiveness we will be eternally condemned. As Dr. David Jeremiah put it, "if you have only been born once, you will have to die twice. But if you have been born twice, you will have to die only once (and you may even escape that one death if Jesus returns to the earth during your lifetime)."[44] If we die physically without being born again we will also die spiritually in hell. When we accept our need for a savior, we are then born again, spiritually. We will only die a physical death and then our soul will live forever in Heaven.

Spiritual Battles

There really is an enemy of our souls who has a plan to kill, steal from, accuse, and destroy us. He has done a good job of fooling us into thinking that he doesn't exist, but he does, and he has one third of all the angels with him to mess us up. The good news is that he has already lost, but he will continue to try to make us ineffective. God has the other two thirds of the angels still with Him, and besides, He created them all anyway, so He can defeat any attack you are facing.

Spiritual Illness

Spiritual illness occurs when we ignore or don't have a relationship with God the Father or when we have accepted Christ as Savior but continue to live in sin. Our thoughts become dark, our words become negative, and our actions become sinful.

Darkness leads to fear, separation, and sadness. One of the hardest things I've ever done—but it brought me significant spiritual growth—was asking God to reveal to me all the sins I had committed for which I hadn't repented. I did this every day until one day there were none. The Bible says we are forgiven when we accept Jesus as our Savior, but that doesn't mean we don't have to fix some of our past mistakes. Each day God revealed anywhere from one to four sins that I had to make right. Some happened so long ago that I had long forgotten them. Some were painful to recall, and as the days went by I would cringe before asking again. At the start I figured a few days to a week would be all. I was wrong. It was around six weeks of daily asking.

Some of the wrongs involved other people, so I had to go apologize or return an item or pay a debt. As hard as it was to humble myself, God was there, and each situation turned out well. Some things I just couldn't make right again, but I did repent, ask God for forgiveness, and ask Him to keep me from repeating those mistakes. God did forgive, and I was set *free!* The Enemy no longer had any dirt on me! I was spotless ... for a while. Slowly but surely, I would get dirty again, but then I would go back to God and be cleansed. I finally realized that if I just asked Him daily it would be easier, so that's what I do now.

The great thing about God is that He chooses to forget our sins when we make things right and ask for His forgiveness. He knew that I needed to be free of bondage even though He also knew it was going to be painful for me. I still remember some of the mistakes I've made, but I'm forgiven, and God has chosen to not remember.

Jeremiah 30:12 tells us, "Your wound is incurable, your injury beyond healing." Verse 15 continues: "Because of your great guilt and many sins I have done these things to you." Then we have the blessing of verse 17: "'But I will restore you to health and heal your wounds,' Declares the LORD."

Don't you see? It's because of our sins that we become sick, but God will forgive and heal us. Here is a list of some possible causes of spiritual Illness:

- Gossiping
- Being unforgiving
- Bitterness
- Breaking any of the Ten Commandments (worshipping false gods; worshipping idols; using God's name wrongly; not honouring the Sabbath; not honouring your parents; committing murder; stealing; lying;

110

committing adultery, which includes thoughts, pornography, etc.; and coveting)

- Breaking laws of your country, region, or city
- Not loving or being loved
- Not having fellowship with others

If we don't follow God, we can expect difficulty. If we do follow God, we can also expect difficulty, so why bother? When we follow God, He gets us through those challenges. Listen to God's promise in Exodus 23:20–26. "I am sending an angel ahead of you to guard you along the way and to bring you to a place I have prepared ... *If* you listen carefully to what he says and do all that I say, I will be an enemy to your enemies and will oppose those who oppose you ... Worship the LORD your God, and His blessing will be on your food and water. I will take away sickness from among you and none will miscarry or be barren in your land. I will give you a full life span" (emphasis mine).

The Bible goes on to say that God would drive out our enemies—but not all at once. God knows that we can only change little by little. The last few verses of the chapter warn against living as the people of the land (our culture) do, because it will lead to sin.

Jesus told a parable of two men who faced storms in life, but one had built on the foundation of God (the rock) and the other on sand (life apart from God). Both faced storms, but the man who had faith in God survived the storm; the one who did not saw his life crumble. What is your foundation?

In 2 Chronicles 26 we read about King Uzziah who "did what was right in the eyes of the Lord ... As long as he sought the Lord, God gave him success ... But after Uzziah became powerful, his *pride* led to his downfall" (emphasis mine). He went into the temple, which was forbidden since he was not a priest. The priests, taking their lives into their hands, confronted Uzziah. He raged at the priests for questioning him. "While he was raging at the priests ... *leprosy* broke out on his forehead" (emphasis mine). It wasn't a coincidence, as "the Lord had afflicted him." He spent the rest of his life in isolation. His son became king, and Uzziah died in disgrace. This warning is especially for leaders in government and business to not let pride cloud our judgment. God puts leaders in place, and He can take them out: "The king's heart is in the hand of the Lord; He directs it like a watercourse wherever He pleases" (Proverbs 21:1).

God outlines things very clearly: Follow Him, and He will protect, provide for, and heal you. Ignore Him, and you will be sick, unprotected, and needy. It's an obvious choice but in North America, Europe, Australia, and other affluent continents, it's easy to think we don't need God. We aren't at "war"; we have all the food we need, and we have a government with dozens of social programs to take care of us.

But look at the promises: no sickness, no miscarriages, long lives, peace, prosperity, protection from those who would oppose us, and love. There are major problems in our world, with only one solution: *repentance*.

Other examples of God causing illness come from Isaiah 37:36, which says, "Then the angel of the lord went out and put to death 185,000 men in the Assyrian camp." Just a few verses later, in 38:4, the Bible tells us, "This is what the Lord, the God of your father David says, 'I have heard your prayer and seen your tears; I will add fifteen years to your life ... And I will defend this city.'"

Here we see both sides of God, the great judge and the healer. God put to death 185,000 men to protect His chosen. These 185,000 were attempting to murder the people of Jerusalem. If God loves us all, why did He kill so many? I don't know, but I trust that God doesn't make mistakes. He doesn't react irrationally. He chose to prevent more unnecessary bloodshed. God had everyone's best interests in mind; He always does.

A few verses later King Hezekiah is near death, so he cries out to God. Through the prophet Isaiah, Hezekiah receives the message that he will be healed and lives another fifteen years! How awesome to know you are healed and will have exactly fifteen more years added to your life. This is divine healing. Not only does Hezekiah receive healing, but he also receives the assurance of protection from invading armies.

God has prepared a place for us. He has sent His angels ahead of us. He is just waiting for us to come. And when He finally gets here, little by little He will change our lives for the better.

Miracles

There are many examples of miraculous healing in the Bible. Exodus 4:6–7 describes God wanting to show Moses the extent of His might; He had Moses put his hand inside his cloak, and when he pulled his hand back out it was leprous. Moses put his hand back in his cloak again, and when he brought it out it was healthy again! God reaffirmed His power by adding, "The Lord said to him [Moses], 'Who gave man his mouth? Who makes him deaf or mute? Who gives him sight or makes him blind? Is it not I, the Lord?'" (Exodus 4:11).

God makes it very clear that He can make sickness and He can heal—instantly.

If you want to read about more miracles of healing, here are some other examples:

- Genesis 20:17
- Exodus 15:26
- 3 John 2
- Psalm 103, in which it is written, "the LORD ...who forgives all your sins and heals all your diseases..."
- Acts 3:6–9, 16; 4:29–31; 5:12–16; 9:32–35; 40–42
- Luke 4:38–41; 7:14–15; 21–22
- Psalm 146:8

There are many more. These are not just stories of old. God

is the same miraculous, healing God today. Call on the name of Jesus Christ, believe, and be healed!

Spiritual Exercises

Pray continually

> If you believe, you will receive whatever you ask for in prayer.
>
> —Matthew 21:22

Read the Bible Daily

Worship God in All Circumstances

Take Care of Widows and Orphans

> Let your light shine before men that they may see your good works and praise your Father in heaven.
>
> —Matthew 5:16

> Trust in the Lord with your whole heart, lean not on your own understanding.
>
> —Proverbs 3:5

Take Risks

> With man this is impossible, but with God all things are possible.
>
> —Matthew 19:26

To paraphrase two other verses, we should also dream big (Genesis 28:15) and look to the future (rather than looking back) (Genesis 19:26).

Seek the Fruit of the Spirit

> But the fruit of the Spirit is love, joy, peace, patience, kindness, goodness, faithfulness, gentleness and self-control.
> —Galatians 5:22

Desire the Gifts of the Spirit

> To one there is given through the Spirit the *message of wisdom*, to another the *message of knowledge* by means of the same Spirit, to another *faith* by the same Spirit, to another *gifts of healing* by that one Spirit, to another *miraculous powers*, to another <u>prophecy</u>, to another *distinguishing between spirits*, to another *speaking in different kinds of tongues*, and to still another the *interpretation of tongues*. All these are the work of one and the same Spirit and He gives them to each one, just as He determines.
> —1 Corinthians 12:8–11, emphasis mine

Listen to God

> The Lord confides in those who fear Him; He makes his covenant known to them.
> —Psalm 25:14

God wants to spend time with us and tell us about our futures. God created us for a special purpose and will tell us what that is when we will spend time with Him. As mentioned earlier, the Bible tells us, "The Lord would speak to Moses face to face, as a man speaks with his friend" (Exodus 33:11). God is not our enemy, but our friend. His is in love with us! You can hear God speaking to you if you take the time to listen. Sometimes God comes as a "gentle whisper": "Then a great and powerful wind tore the mountains apart and shattered the rocks before the Lord, but the Lord was not in the wind. After the wind there was an earthquake, but the Lord was not in the earthquake. After the earthquake came a fire, but the Lord was not in the fire. And after the fire came a gentle whisper" (1 Kings 19:11–13).

As the previous quotation illustrates, God comes after difficulty to comfort us. But we don't have to wait for disaster; we can listen to God's whisper today! You have to find a quiet place and listen. Sometimes it helps to be in nature. I would start by asking, "Lord, are you there?" "Yes, I am," will be his reply. Gradually I started asking other questions. At first I thought I was just hearing my own thoughts, because the voice was only in my mind. Gradually I realized that it was not my voice but God's. You can tell it is God by the answers. He always tells the truth. Ask a question that you know God will answer a certain way. For example, "God, do you love me?" The answer will always be yes. Other questions to ask are, "Who will I become? What do you want me to know? What do you want me to do? What do you want me to enjoy? What do you want me to change? Are there any sins I've committed that I need to repent of?" You can think of others. Those are the questions I usually ask on a daily basis.

God wants to speak to you as a person speaks with a friend, so spend time getting to know God as your best friend. He is always there and always ready to listen. It has been documented that we become more like those people we spend time with. The more time we spend with God the godlier we will become.

If you do these things then you will experience the God of the universe. You will live the victorious, exciting, supernatural life you were created for.

In the next chapter you will learn one of the most misunderstood and probably the most overlooked aspect of health.

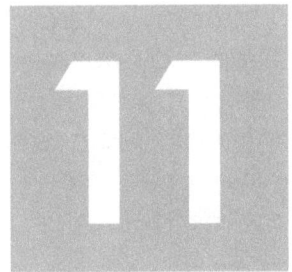

Nerve Function

"The eye is the lamp of the body. If your eyes are healthy, your whole body will be full of light."
—Matthew 6:22

The nervous system controls and coordinates <u>all</u> the organs and structures of the human body.
—Gray's Anatomy
(emphasis mine)

The human nervous system is comprised of the brain, spinal cord, and trillions of nerve cells called neurons. It is the first system to form after conception, and it is the master controller of all the other organs and tissues in the body. The nervous system is responsible for relating us to our environment and maintaining homeostasis or balance in our bodies. The term chiropractors coined over a hundred years ago to describe this intricate balance is "innate intelligence." In other words, our bodies know best what to do to keep us as healthy as possible, given the current conditions.

When old cells die, the nervous system signals the body to generate a new cell. The body does not recycle old dead cells; it makes new ones. If it did recycle, we wouldn't have to continually eat. Our skin is only a few weeks old. Did you know that over 90 percent of house dust is made up of dead human skin cells? When you vacuum or dust your house you are actually cleaning yourself and your family off the furniture!

Every day old cells die and new ones are made. This only

happens if there is a signal from the nervous system. Literally every day, we become a new creation. Every day our hair and fingernails grow. We keep cutting them off, and they keep growing. Our red blood cells are continually replaced roughly every thirty days. We have a new liver every month also. Our skeleton is only ten years old.[45] How miraculous!

Not every system in our bodies is continually replaced. There is one system that is not: the nervous system. The nervous system is responsible for controlling all of the body's systems. It is broken down into two main systems: the autonomic nervous system and the voluntary nervous system. When we talk about *reflexes*, we're referring to the automatic system. Roughly 90 percent of what our bodies do is because of our reflexes. We have reflexes in our muscles, our eyes, and our internal organs. Essentially everything that is not voluntarily controlled is automatic and, therefore, a reflex. We don't voluntarily digest food; our brains automatically control that. The same goes for breathing, immunity, reproduction, circulation, and so on.

Some systems have dual control. For example, we can take a deep breath at any time or hold our breath. If we hold it for too long, we pass out, our innate intelligence (brain) takes over, and we start breathing again. Posture is mainly automatic, but it has some voluntary control also.

When most people think of nerves, they often think of pain. When nerves get pinched, compressed, over stretched, irritated, or inflamed, they will hurt. However, there is no pain most of the time when nerves malfunction. Only about 10 percent of our nerves are for pain. So a person can experience nerve malfunction but not have any pain associated with it.

Nerves and Cancer

Nerves are what tell our brains what is happening in the body, and then the brain tells the body what to do. If the nervous system is not functioning properly, the immune system will malfunction. When this happens, cancer cells will start to multiply. According to cancer specialist Dr. Yoshimizu, our bodies make three thousand to six thousand new cancer cells daily! If the immune system is working, they are killed and a person never gets sick. However, if the immune system is weak, the cancer cells will grow. He says that it takes nine to fourteen years for the tumor to grow to a one-centimeter mass. It then takes another three years for it to become one kilogram or ten centimeters. By then, most people are nearing death.

Dr. Yoshimizu has observed that people who go to chiropractors are more likely to survive cancer than people who don't. This is because the nervous system controls the immune system. When nerves are compressed or irritated, they don't function properly, which impairs the function of the immune system and other organs.

Many times people think that reflexes are bad. Most people don't see coughing as a blessing, but coughing is actually a good thing. It is a reflex (your body's innate intelligence) attempting to get something out that is bad. Cough suppressants allow the infection to remain and go deeper into the lungs, leading to worse infections, such as pneumonia. It's even worse than that, however: some children die from the drugs used to stop coughing.[46]

If the body didn't have natural ways to get rid of infections, life would be very short. Sneezing, vomiting, and diarrhea are other ways the body rids itself of toxins. Let it happen. Remember: toxicity is one of the three causes of illness.

As our bodies heal, we may experience these reflexes in an unpleasant way. What we perceive as the illness is actually our bodies ridding us of the illness. These symptoms are not the problem; symptoms mean our bodies are getting rid of the problem or letting us know we have a problem. For example, a fever is a symptom of infection. Our bodies generate the fever to kill off the bad bacteria or virus. It is *not* the infection that creates the fever; it is the body. This is very important to understand because if we stop our bodies from doing what is best for us (even if it doesn't feel good), we will *assist* the disease. The fever is generated to kill the germ. So in other words, a fever is a good thing. It is our innate intelligence protecting us. Taking a drug to suppress a fever allows the infection to continue, which means it takes longer for the body to heal.

Taking drugs, whether they are legal, illegal, prescription, or over the counter will usually inhibit our bodies from healing. Our innate intelligence is always trying to get us healthy again. Our bodies never do anything bad for us. It might not feel good, but it is what we need to regain health. So taking drugs not only stops our bodies from healing, but it also creates a new problem: toxicity. Drug companies like to call this "side effects." It doesn't sound as bad that way, but it is bad. Not only is the original problem still there but now you have toxic chemicals in your system.

There are no safe drugs on the market. Every drug is a poison. In small amounts it may have some symptomatic benefit, but in larger amounts or with continuous use it kills people. The third and fourth leading causes of *preventable* deaths in the US are essentially drug use. According to Barbara Starfield MD, MPH, every year roughly 119,000 people die from medical negligence or errors, and 106,000 people die from taking "correctly administered medications."[47] Use drugs only in life or death situations, or they could be the death of you.

Now I know some of you are thinking that drugs have been responsible for some "miraculous" recoveries. Maybe this has been true for you or someone you know. If it was miraculous, it wasn't a drug: it was God. Certainly drugs have helped people, but most of the time they could have been avoided. For example, high blood pressure is caused by one or a combination of the following factors: emotional stress, poor diet, chronic dehydration, improper breathing, smoking, lack of exercise, and spinal misalignment. These are the only causes that have any credible scientific evidence. It's not due to a lack of pills. Yes, drugs can bring a person's blood pressure down, but are they healthier than removing the causes of the problem? No. As you just read, 106,000 people per year die in the US from taking drugs as medically directed; what about the rest of the world? It's probably a million people every year! So follow the principles in this book, and you won't be sick or taking drugs. Every disease has a cause, and the cause is not a lack of drugs.

As our bodies heal, we may experience new symptoms, called *recovery symptoms*, or re-experience old symptoms, a process called *retracing*. Recovery symptoms are usually described as a "cold" or are compared to the flu. As our bodies heal and toxins are eliminated, we might actually feel sick. It is a good sign. Let it happen without taking some drug. Drink lots of water and really watch what you are eating. You may have headaches, low energy, or diarrhea. You might experience a sudden increase in energy or euphoria. All of these are normal.

Retracing is a little different from having recovery symptoms. It can come in the form of pain in areas that were previously painful but have been pain free for some time. For example, you may have injured your knee a year ago, but the pain went away. Now that you are working on your health and your body is changing, the knee pain could flare up. Emotional retracing happens when you experience flashbacks or in some cases crying, laughter, or strange dreams. Retracing can come in a variety of symptoms, so don't become worried and run back to medicating the symptoms. You will only have to deal with it again in the future if you want to fully heal. Taking a medication stops the healing process, as we have already discussed. You may feel better temporarily, but you will have to go back and deal with it again eventually. Just deal with it right away, and then you can move on. Taking something to deal with symptoms is like getting drunk to forget sorrows. The alcohol may numb the emotional pain but when it wears off the problem is still there plus a hangover.

Nerves

Nerves are the highways along which the brain transmits and receives information to and from the body. This is constant two-way communication. For example, when you eat, food travels down to the stomach, which sends a signal back to brain to make digestion happen. When you are full, your brain tells you that you are full. Meanwhile digestion continues passing the food into the intestine until eventually it passes out of the body. All along the digestive tract the brain transmits and receives information, even though we are not consciously aware of it.

Subluxations

The term coined by chiropractic doctors over one hundred years ago to describe interference to our bodies' innate intelligence is *subluxation*. Subluxations can be caused by physical, chemical, emotional, or spiritual stress.

Physical Stress

Physical stress can come in the form of a sudden trauma (macro trauma) or repeated trauma (micro trauma). Common causes are whiplash, motor vehicle collisions, falls, sports injuries (sprain, strains), workplace injuries, or blows to the body. Many of these happen in childhood. Also, the birth process is a common source of physical trauma. Children are especially susceptible to subluxations if they were born by cesarean section or if their births were aided by forceps or vacuum extraction. These can lead to severe compression of the spinal cord and blood vessels to the brain, which can cause sudden infant death syndrome (SIDS).

Chemical Stress

Chemical stress comes from air pollution, smoking, breathing toxins, drinking unhealthy things (fluoride, sugar, caffeine, etc.), eating unhealthy things (trans fats, soy oil, fast food, etc.), and putting things on our bodies that are toxic (sunscreen, deodorants, makeup, etc.). When a person smokes, he or she causes stress to the lungs, which signals the brain with a warning about the stress. This causes a reflex tightening of the muscles around the spine that the nerves of the lungs go to (upper back). Gradually this causes more tension, lack of motion, and pulling on the spine, which leads to compensation. Improper motion or misalignment leads to abnormal wear and tear.

Emotional Stress

Emotional stress comes from abnormal emotional stress over time. Someone who is constantly angry, sad, or upset will be constantly stressed. We can all look at a person and tell if he or she is angry. The person's body language says it all. Tight fists, tense shoulders, clenched jaw, and furled brow all communicate anger. Unreleased emotion causes a stress pattern. This abnormal tension creates an abnormal posture, which leads to subluxations. A person almost always has multiple layers of emotional stress patterns. In fact, I have come to realize that the majority of health problems in adults today are from past emotional stresses. Many of these stresses happen in childhood and are not properly corrected or handled. For example, the children of a divorce are often not able to deal with their emotional issues because both parents are emotionally unwell. I have found the chiropractic technique of KST (Koren Specific Technique) to work really well in dealing with emotional stress.

Spiritual Stress

Spiritual stress comes from not having a right relationship with God. Fear of judgment or death, guilt from wrongdoing (illegal music downloads, cheating on taxes, speeding, etc.), or going against God's will (viewing pornography, swearing, not spending time with God, and breaking any of the commandments) are examples of spiritual stresses. For example, studies show that bitterness or unforgiveness leads to illnesses, such as cancer. Choosing not to forgive people will literally make you sick. Forgiving someone that has done something wrong does not mean that you are saying that what the person did was acceptable; you are just choosing to accept that he or she made a mistake, and you are going to move on with your life. Unforgiveness is like taking a poison and thinking that it will make the other person sick. Phone the person if possible or write a letter informing the person that you forgive him or her.

These spiritual stresses increase stress hormone levels, which weaken a person's health and can literally cause cancer.

In addition to these nervous system problems, we can also get biomechanical problems.

Arthritis

Most people falsely believe that arthritis is just part of getting older, which is not true. I have seen x-rays of older people who don't have arthritis, and I've seen it in children. There are different types of arthritis. The most common form is osteoarthritis (OA). According to the American Arthritis Foundation, 27 million Americans have arthritis.[48] Other authors claim that 100 percent of people seventy years old and above will have some form of arthritis.

Essentially, arthritis is damage to joints. There are different causes of OA, but usually it's caused by *abnormal* wear and tear or injuries. Whiplash, for example, causes damage to

124

the cartilage in the neck and spine, which leads to arthritis. When joints are not properly aligned, they endure abnormal stress and wear out, just like gears that grind together. Healthy joints don't wear out. According to whiplash expert Dr. Arthur Croft, normal joints have the same amount of friction as ice on ice and will not wear out. But when joints are misaligned or subluxated, they start to wear out.

Even a lack of motion causes joints to become unhealthy. Just like muscles that are not being used, cartilage will atrophy if it is not being exercised. Sitting around hoping not to wear out will cause you to weaken. I would highly recommend going to a chiropractor and taking care of your joints and nerves.

Unfortunately not every doctor of chiropractic can help you reverse arthritis. Some might claim they can, but unless they have x-rays to prove it, how would they know? Pettibon chiropractors (and others) take x-rays to determine your initial condition and then check later to see if you are improving. Restoring the discs, alignment, and motion in joints will allow the body to heal so that arthritis can be stopped and eventually reversed. The process of losing the space and the cartilage deteriorating is osteoarthritis or spinal decay. We have a protocol in my office that can stop arthritis from progressing and if caught early enough, reverse it.

Phase one spinal decay starts with the normal position and function of the spine being compromised. The discs become squished and stressed due to abnormal wear and tear. This can lead to disc bulging, compression, or herniation. Most likely, nerves will either be compressed, pinched, or irritated. As nerves get compressed or irritated, they malfunction, leading to a whole host of health issues. This causes a vicious cycle that inhibits the body from being able to heal itself.

If uncorrected, the joints continue to deteriorate, leading to loss of height, more stiffness, loss of motion, and more nerve damage and pain.

In phase two there are now obvious changes to the bones, which are commonly referred to as bone spurs. These can rub on delicate soft tissues, such as blood vessels, nerves, ligaments, tendons, or muscles.

The third phase is characterized by almost a complete loss of disc material and significant health problems, constant pain, and poor posture. Think of little old people who are hunched over and obviously not very mobile. These people will generally be using a cane, walker, or wheelchair.

The final phase is almost complete joint destruction and bone on bone. Most people don't live very long when they are in this phase because of the nerve damage impairing cell function. When nerves die, cells and tissues die. This phase is very unlikely to improve fully, but some improvement is possible.

The first three phases are usually reversible. Most people can get back to normal if they start working on their problems while in phase one. By time the joints are at phase two, they are not likely to get back to 100 percent. They usually can get back to phase one. When treatment starts during phase three, people will usually get back to phase two. The sooner you catch the problem, the better. The longer a joint is subluxated, the worse it becomes and the harder it is to heal.

Prevention is the key; don't wait until your health is really bad to go to a chiropractor. If you wait until you have chronic pain, you will probably find that you will are already in phase two. Research shows that by age thirteen, one out of every three children (33 percent) already have observable joint and disc damage on an MRI. Most of those don't even know it because they aren't in pain, but if left uncorrected the damage will create health problems as the children get older.[49] Anywhere from 56 percent to 72 percent of twenty-one year olds with no back pain will have disc degeneration on MRI.[50] By time we are forty years old most of us will have had at least one bout of back pain, unless we are actively preventing the disc decay by getting regular chiropractic care.

No Pain, No Problem

It's possible to have nerve compression in the spine and not get spinal pain, but there can be pain in the extremities (arms or legs) or other symptoms, such as constipation, allergies, asthma, fatigue, poor immune system, headaches, skin problems, bed wetting, dizziness, ringing in the ears, or impotency, just to name a few.

Most people don't wait until they have rotten teeth to go to a dentist; why not treat your spine the same and get it checked before you are sick and hurting? While you're at it, get your kids and/or grandkids checked also.

One of the worst measures of a person's health is pain or an absence of it. There are many health issues that are not painful. For example, high blood pressure, diabetes, weight gain, clogged arteries, thin bones (osteoporosis), tooth decay, low thyroid hormone, high stress hormone, nerve pressure, and others. Remember that there are three phases to health: healthy, unhealthy, or sick. When a person is not healthy, he or she can have clogging arteries but not realize it until the heart attack. The same is true with nerves: pressure can cause vital-organ malfunction while a person remains pain free until there is severe compression or inflammation.

I have experienced this firsthand. I used to have horrible spring hay fever allergies. It wasn't painful, but it was certainly horrible. Through chiropractic care I no longer suffer from allergies. The problem was nerve compression in my neck, yet it didn't hurt.

Pain doesn't usually manifest until the problem is really bad. Even in extreme situations, such as a car crash, research has shown that it can be several days before a person feels pain or at least until the person fully feels the effects of the injury.

Don't be fooled into thinking that if you don't have pain, your health is 100 percent. You may have nerve compression, clogged arteries, or other issues that will get worse if not treated. Don't wait until you have rotten teeth to see a dentist, and don't wait until you have pain to see a chiropractor. You will save yourself time, money, and suffering it you are proactive.

Earthing

God put the first people on the earth in a garden, not a city. They lived in a warm climate, so they either walked around barefoot or with sandals made from animal skins (leather). In the last one hundred years, shoes have gone from being leather to rubber soled. We are now *disconnected from the earth*. Research shows that we need to be connected to the earth to dissipate free radicals from our bodies.

Touching the earth with our bare skin literally grounds us. If electronics are not grounded, they can build up abnormal electrical charges that lead to short-circuiting. People also need to touch the earth to decrease the stress of living in an electronic world of cell phones, Wi-Fi, high-voltage power lines, and electrical currents everywhere. This would not be so bad if we walked around grounded, but we don't.

Most people recognize that they feel better if they walk barefoot on the grass or on the beach. There is research to show that it improves our stress hormone levels to connect to the earth. Maybe that is why some people love to garden; they are de-stressing in a mental sense and in an electrical sense too.

In the next chapter we explore the microscopic world of bacteria and viruses and why you don't need to be afraid of them.

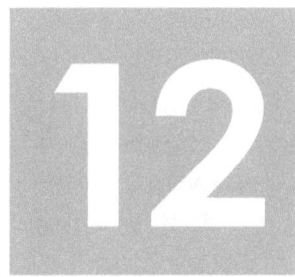

Germs

> But the Pharisee, noticing that Jesus did not first
> wash before the meal, was surprised.
> —Luke 11:38

People think that germs cause illness, but the reality is they can only live in an environment that is suitable for them. Germs are like seeds: they need the right conditions to grow and thrive. The odds of a handful of carrot seeds growing in your pocket are pretty slim. But if I were to put the seeds in some soil with water and adequate warmth and sunlight and air, I would expect those seeds would grow. So it is with microorganisms (germs): just because they are on our bodies or in our bodies doesn't mean that they will grow. Germs *cannot* make a healthy person sick all on their own; we have an immune system that was created to defend us from these unseen invaders.

None of these germs are new either. Genesis 1 says God created all things, so that would include microscopic organisms. We were designed to be able to fend bad germs off, but not all germs are bad. There are good ones as well as bad, and we need germs to be healthy.

What most people perceive as diseases are actually the symptoms of a disease that the body is attempting to get rid of. If you have a fever, as discussed previously, don't treat it. If you want to sanitize your dishes, wash them in hot water. Heat kills bad germs on dishes and in the body. Many people who die from infections die not from the infection but from the medications given to treat it. When a drug decreases the fever, the body's defenses are weakened. Sure, a person "feels better," but is he or she healthier? No! The problem is still there, but now it's going to be harder to get rid of it. Your body wants you to stay alive, so it is going to do whatever it has to make sure that you get better. The less you interfere, the better. Your body will never do anything that is harmful to you. After all, we would all die moments after birth if our bodies wanted us dead. You might be asking yourself, "What about autoimmune diseases? Isn't the body attacking itself?" It is, but just bear with me for a moment, and I will explain why.

Right now the microscopic organisms on our bodies outnumber the cells that make up our bodies. There are ten times more bacteria in us and on us than there are human cells. The vast majority of them are beneficial, but some are harmful. The helpful ones are called "probiotics." Without probiotics we would not be able to properly digest food or fight off all the so-called bad germs.

We are all covered by germs from the moment we are born. When a baby is born, his or her mouth is usually facing down, or toward the mother's bottom. As the baby passes through the birth canal, he or she is exposed to thousands of vaginal microorganisms and then to even more germs as his or her head pushes out a little bit of feces from Mom's rectum. This feces has bacteria in it; through this action, the bacteria are introduced to the baby. When baby breast-feeds for the very first time, he or she ingests even more germs that are on Mom's skin.

If it weren't for germs we would not have cheese, yogurt, sour cream, sauerkraut, balsamic vinegar, or wine.

Many people today are fearful of germs. They carry around hand sanitizers, they are constantly washing, and they worry when they hear someone cough or sneeze. Jesus was not afraid of germs. Luke 11:38 says, "The Pharisee, noticing that Jesus did not first wash before the meal, was surprised." The Pharisee was surprised because it was social etiquette to wash and part of Jewish law. Jesus was showing the man that even if we look clean on the outside, we could still be sinful on the inside. I think Jesus was also showing us that we don't need to live in fear of germs. As I mentioned earlier, there are good and bad germs, both of which are killed off when we wash. Harsh detergents or products containing chemicals for colour and fragrance in cleaning products are most likely harming our health.

Many health officials warn against the use of soaps containing antibiotics. It's not necessary to use antibiotics every time a person washes, and the bacteria are becoming resistant to the antibiotics. This has helped create a whole new strain of "superbugs." The indiscriminant use of antibiotics for ear and upper respiratory infections is also part of the problem. Most of these infections are from viruses; antibiotics only kill bacteria. Antibiotics not only kill bad germs but good ones also. Using antibiotics is kind of like using a bomb to get rid of the enemy army in your city. Sure the enemy will be dead, but so will all the good people.

Antibiotics are not safe. They cause harm, especially to the digestive system. If you have ever taken any antibiotics, it's crucial that you get some probiotics. Farmers use antibiotics to fatten up their animals. Antibiotics that kill a type of bacteria called H. pylori in the stomach lead to overeating. People with low levels of H. pylori have lower levels of an appetite-suppressing hormone, so these people tend to be overeaters. Who would have thought that bacteria could keep us from eating too much?[51]

Children born by cesarean section have higher rates of asthma and allergies. It appears that vaginal bacteria have a role to play in developing a properly functioning immune system. If that's not bad enough, consider that 40 percent of children who receive a broad-spectrum antibiotic will suffer from severe diarrhea due to disturbing the normal bacteria in the body.[52] The Centers for Disease Control report on their website that "studies have shown that 30-50% of antibiotics prescribed in hospitals are unnecessary or incorrect."[53] Many childhood diseases are actually beneficial and help to build up our immune system so we don't get sick as adults. It is a normal part of development for children to get sick.

Autoimmune disorders

The rates of autism, Alzheimer's disease, dementia, autoimmune disorders, attention deficit disorders, and other illnesses have been steadily increasing. Some autoimmune disorders appear to be linked to environmental toxins, moulds, drug resistant bacteria, chemicals and drugs. Some chemicals (toxins) mimic our own hormones which then disrupts normal body functions. If these substances get into our cells then the body doesn't recognize it as self so it directs the immune system to attack it. Some toxins build up in certain tissues, such as the joints, so the body attacks the cells in the joints. Most people then think that the body is attacking itself, but in reality it's attacking the abnormal cells or toxins. Obviously we wouldn't survive very long if our body was attacking itself. There must be an underlying cause for the immune system to malfunction.

There is a better way. Get healthy! Healthy people can survive germ outbreaks. Healthy people don't get colds and flus. When a person is healthy, his or her immune system is working at 100 percent and can fight off any illness. Why didn't everyone die of the bubonic plague? The people out carting off dead bodies survived because they had healthy immune systems. Everyone was exposed to the bubonic plague, but about a third of the people never became sick.

On June 11, 2009 the World Health Organization reported that the influenza (H1N1) pandemic of 2009 had affected 70 of the 195 countries around the world. That's only thirty six percent of the countries on earth and most of those countries were the most wealthy (US, Canada, England, etc.) In other words, seventy four percent of the countries around the world did not have a significant outbreak of the H1N1 flu. The Centers for Disease Control and Prevention in the United States, published a report that *"estimated* that at least 1 million cases of 2009 H1N1 influenza had occurred in the United States."* (emphasis mine). The United States Census Bureau reported the population in 2009 to be 306.8 million people. That is only 0.3 percent (three out of every one thousand) of the population getting sick from H1N1. So 99.7 percent of the population did not get sick. I remember all the fear, the hype and propaganda used to get people to take unnecessary drugs and shots. The H1N1 vaccination program did not even began until October 2009. By then the so called outbreak was already basically over. The CDC also reported that the vast majority of people who became sick were obese.[54]

The underlying problem is most people are not healthy enough to fight off these germs because they are not living well. They are not living the way to optimal health that I am outlining in this book, so it is no surprise that they are going to get sick. It is not a matter of *if*, just *when*. So the fear sets in that illness is lurking around the corner, and most of us feel better when we do something proactive.

We can't get a shot and then just carry on with a lifestyle that leads to sickness. There is no magic pill that will keep a person healthy if they are full of toxins and deficient in nutrients. There is no quick fix to health. The main reason why these infections are rare today in developed countries is that we know about sanitation, hand washing, clean water, proper food handling, cooking, and refrigeration. For example, many bacteria are spread from mouth to mouth or from feces to mouth. In other words, not washing after going to the bathroom or handling food with dirty hands could spread unhealthy bacteria from someone who is infected to someone who isn't. Obviously the solution is simple, wash after going to the bathroom.

The good news is our bodies have the ability to fight foreign invaders. We just need to provide ourselves with necessary nutrients and remove any deficiency so that our bodies can function properly. These germs have been around since God created everything (see Genesis 1). There are no new bugs, animals, plants, or other life forms on our planet. There are fewer life forms than there once were, in fact, due to extinction. We just didn't know that these microscopic life forms were there until about two hundred years ago.

Due to drugs and other chemicals some microorganisms have mutated. We now have antibiotic resistant bacteria or superbugs. Polio was a disease that began in Canada, the United States and Sweden after the introduction of pesticides. This was not and is still not a disease of poor underdeveloped countries. The name polio has been replaced by meningitis in most developed countries now which makes tracking the incidence of it challenging.

In 1948 Dr. Benjamin Sandler a nutritional expert at the Oteen Veterans' Hospital reported a link between polio and sugar consumption. He found that the countries with the highest per capita consumption of sugar, such as Australia, Britain, Canada, Sweden and the United States had the greatest incidence of polio. In contrast, polio was practically unheard of in China where sugar use was ninety seven per cent less per capita.

Researchers had noticed for years that polio rates spiked during the summer months. He presumed that sugar consumption also increased in summer so in 1949 he warned residents of North Carolina to decrease consumption of ice cream, soft drinks and other high sugar foods. That summer the people of North Carolina decreased their consumption of sugar by 90 percent and the number of polio infections decreased by the same amount. The North Carolina State Health department reported only 229 cases of polio in 1949 compared to the 2,498 from the previous year. Sadly due to heavy marketing from the companies affected by the downturn in their sales people returned to eating more sugar and by the summer of 1950 the number of polio cases was back up to "normal" levels again.[55]

Many people foolishly think that with vaccines, many bacteria or viruses will be eliminated. How can you destroy something that is microscopic and has been around for thousands of years? It only takes one bacterium to start an epidemic. Even the late Louis Pasteur, who was one of the first to discover microorganisms, said that "host resistance" is the key to preventing infections.

Everyone on the planet has essentially all the same germs in them and on them. So why is there an Ebola outbreak in West Africa or a measles outbreak in Canada? The short answer is the people there aren't healthy. When a person's immune system can't deal with some of these bad germs, he or she gets sick. Many people have been exposed to Ebola, measles, the bubonic plague, or HIV and never become ill. As I have mentioned in the previous chapter, nerve malfunction, stresses and lifestyle factors come into play. We are all carriers of germs that can make us sick, but not all of us get sick.

We always have and always will need microorganisms to help our body function properly. The question is not, "What can I do to avoid germs?" It is, "What do I need to do to be healthy enough to fight the unhealthy germs?" Hopefully, you are better able to answer that question as you have been reading this book. But we are not done yet there are still a couple factors left to discuss about the way to getting healthy.

Unfortunately, some people are born with genetic problems that will affect their health, which is the focus of the next chapter.

Genetics

For you formed my inward parts; You weaved me in my mother's womb. I will give thanks to Thee for I am fearfully and wonderfully made; Wonderful are thy works, and my soul knows it very well. My frame was not hidden from Thee, when I was made in secret, and skillfully wrought in the depths of the earth.

—Psalm 139:13–15

Did you know that the DNA strands in each cell of our bodies are compacted seven thousand times smaller than their actual size? Each strand of DNA measures seven centimeters on its own, but when inside a cell it only measures ten microns (or 0.01 millimeters). This would be like taking something that is as long as your finger and making it microscopic. How amazing! How wonderful! DNA is the heart of our cells, the structure that determines how our bodies function. If all our DNA were stretched out end to end, they would measure 5.3 billion kilometers long!

Our genes are the blueprints for our cells. In essence, our genes tell our cells what proteins to make. Most of us are born with healthy genes; the ones who aren't usually demonstrate it right at birth. For example, Down syndrome (trisomy 21) children are born with an extra twenty-first chromosome. It is obvious by their facial features that something is not right immediately at birth. There is nothing that can be done to change this. The cause is not fully known but is most likely due to toxicity during or before pregnancy. Certain chemicals will alter genetic structure and function.

I want to be clear that some genetic changes can lead to severe illness whereas others do not. A person can still work on optimizing their health even if they are born with Down syndrome or some other genetic condition. A genetic condition does not make a person any less beautiful or worthy. If the genetic condition affects that person's optimal function in some way then they will not be healthy by the definition I am using. However, that person can follow the information contained in this book and be as healthy as possible.

Only about 1 to 5 percent of human illness can be directly and solely attributed to genetic causes. In such cases the genes are altered, and there is nothing that can be done to change them.

According to the World Health Organization (WHO), cancer is *not* a genetic disorder. Cancer occurs because of genetic mutations that affect the cells' ability to multiply and repair. These mutations happen because of toxicity and/or deficiency. It takes around twenty years to develop cancer. According to the WHO, "Tumors enlarge because cancer cells lack the ability to balance cell division and cell death and by forming their own vascular system (blood supply)."[56]

The WHO goes on to state, "Studies have shown that the primary determinants of most cancers are *lifestyle factors*, such as tobacco, dietary and exercise habits, environmental carcinogens and infectious agents, rather than inherited genetic factors. In fact, the proportion of cancers caused by high penetrance genes is low, about *less than 5%* for breast cancer and less for most other cancer types except retinoblastoma in children" (emphasis mine).

What they are saying is over 95 percent of all cancers are caused by our choices. To smoke or not, to exercise regularly or not, to eat well or not—these are all choices we make. We can't blame our parents or grandparents, because there could be abnormal genes in all of us; if we live well, we won't become sick. My maternal grandmother died of breast cancer in her early forties, but my mother is still alive and is in her seventies, even though she is carrying the "breast cancer gene". If cancer were a purely genetic problem, she would be dead by now.

In fact, the best studies that show that cancer is not genetic come from studying identical twins. Identical twins don't simply look identical; they have the exact same genes. Many studies show one twin getting a cancer that the other does not. If cancer and other types of illness were genetic, both twins would get them in the same place and on the same day. This doesn't happen. Genetic illnesses are hardwired into the system. In other words, there is nothing you can do to cause or prevent them. Genetic illness is like eye colour: there is nothing you can do to choose it or change it.

Many people think of aging as a disease, but this is not true either. Most scientists think we are genetically programmed to live for 120 years and as I mentioned earlier that is what God said in Genesis chapter 20. Our cells don't live for 120 years and then all die at once. Our cells are constantly being replaced. Old cells die and new ones are made. For example, our red blood cells only live for thirty days, and then they are genetically programmed to die. New ones are constantly being made to replace the old cells in our blood and in every other tissue. If a person is not living according to his or her genetic requirements, the rate of cell death will speed up and a person will die sooner than the 120 years we are programmed to live.

It's obvious that most people aren't living congruently with their genes, because the average lifespan is only eighty years. Basically what's happening is most people's lifestyles are causing them to age faster and die sooner than they should. Not exercising, eating unhealthy food, smoking, stress, subluxations, and all the other toxins and deficiencies that I've discussed so far cause us to become sick and die younger than we should.

The study of epigenetics has shed a lot of light on this subject. Our genes tell our cells what proteins to make through a series of on/off switches. Every cell in our bodies has the same genes, but some cells are blood cells, some are brain cells, and so on. The reason we don't grow eyes on the backs of our heads is the on/off switches.

When old cells die our bodies will create new ones. If there is some miscommunication, a cell can become something other than what it was intended to be. There are many chemicals in food and the environment now that affect these on/off switches, leading to malfunctioning cells. Having too many malfunctioning cells causes organs to work improperly.

Scientific research has shown that if we don't exercise, our genes cannot function properly. Our bodies start to malfunction and break down because we were designed to be active, not sedentary. If we don't exercise for two days, our cells start to suffer, we get weaker, and we lose cell function. However, as soon as we start to exercise, our genes start to function properly again.

A 2008 study on twenty-four hundred identical twins was very clear: people who exercise moderately for one hundred minutes per week (fifteen minutes per day) had genes (telomeres) that looked like someone five to six years younger than someone who only exercised sixteen minutes per week. Those people who exercised three hours per week (thirty minutes per day) genetically appeared to be about nine years younger than the sedentary group. The more people exercised, the healthier their genes were; the overall health of the individuals increased as well. Conversely, people who are sedentary age more rapidly, get sicker, and die younger.[57]

The same thing happens if we eat too many grains, processed foods, sugars, or other toxins; as soon as we start to eat congruently with our genetics, we get healthier.

Toxic thoughts can have the same effect on our genes. Negativity and unhealthy thoughts cause stress, and stress hormones at too high a level for too long will cause genetic maladaptation.

Poor health is usually not a genetic problem; it is just the symptom of poor lifestyle. It is easier to blame our poor choices on our genes than to take ownership of our poor or uninformed choices. Don't fall into the trap of believing that there is nothing you can do. You are not a drug company slave. You don't have the obesity gene or the diabetes gene or the "I can't speak in public" gene or the "I can't do math" gene. You have the potential to be great; believe it.

In the next and final chapter I will tie all of these concepts together and give you most important key to optimal health.

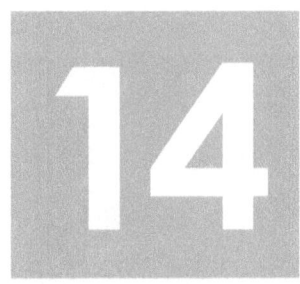

The Most Important Key to Health

Do you remember the quiz from chapter 1? Go back and read that chapter if you haven't yet. I have included the quiz here with the answers and/or helpful explanatory information. Hopefully these answers and facts will be familiar by now.

Define Healthy

Healthy is defined as having a body, mind, and spirit that are 100 percent functional; healthy is not just the absence of disease.

What Are the Thirteen Factors You Need to Be Healthy?

The thirteen factors you need to be healthy are the subjects of this book's latter thirteen chapters: sunlight (chapter 2), clean water (chapter 3), healthy food (chapter 4), exercise (chapter 5), sleep (chapter 6), fresh air (chapter 7), mental attitude (chapter 8), good hygiene (chapter 9), spiritual health (chapter 10), proper nerve function (chapter 11), germs (chapter 12), proper gene function (chapter 13), and the most important key to health (chapter 14)—which I explain later in this chapter.

Are You Tired at the End of Your Workday?

If your job is not a very strenuous one, you shouldn't be tired at the end of your workday. If you have a sedentary job you will probably feel tired from a lack of motion. Get yourself a Wobble Chair or other active sitting chair or a stand up work station.

Do You Nap?

If you are getting proper sleep and are healthy, you don't need to nap.

Do You Get at Least One Cold Each Year?

Healthy people don't get colds.

Are Your Blood Pressure and Resting Heart Rate Too High?

Your resting blood pressure should be under 120 over 80, and your resting heart rate should be around sixty beats per minute. Emotional stress, smoking, lack of exercise, poor diet and nerve compression can cause blood pressure to go up. Medication is rarely necessary when you address those factors.

Do You Run Out of Air in Under Thirty Seconds When Holding Your Breath?

You should be able to hold your breath for at least thirty seconds at rest. If not you should be exercising and getting adjustments to help with lung function.

Are You Performing the Four Different Types of Exercise That You Need Inconsistently or Less Than Daily?

Every day you should perform postural, stretching, strengthening, and aerobic exercises.

Do You Smoke?

Smoking is detrimental to good health and is bad for more than just the lungs. Smoking anything is unhealthy, this includes cigarettes, cigars and marijuana.

Do You Drink Less Than Two Liters of Water in a Day?

The average adult needs to drink at least two litres (8 cups) of water per day. Do not drink coffee daily or juice (except for that which has been freshly juiced), but herbal tea is acceptable. If you want to drink coffee make sure to drink organic coffee only. Only drink cold fluids when you are really hot, most of the time drink warm or room temperature liquids. Adding fresh lemon or lime juice will make water healthier and be sure you are getting enough minerals/electrolytes from sea salt or Himalayan salt.

Do you drink pop daily?

Any soda pop is unhealthy, especially diet pop. A healthy option is to drink carbonated mineral water with some lemon or lime added to it.

Is Your Diet Low in Omega-3 Fatty Acids?

Omega-3 fatty acids come from fish and other sources. Unless you want to eat fish daily, you will need a supplement. Take roughly a quarter teaspoon for every twenty pounds of body weight. Confirm your requirement with a health professional who has nutritional training (usually not a medical doctor).

Do You Eat Less Than Seven Servings of Fruits and Vegetables Daily?

Eat at least seven servings of fruits and vegetables daily, not including rice, grains, or corn. When possible eat local, fresh and non-genetically modified plants. In the colder months be sure to eat more cooked vegetables. Be careful that they are not overcooked.

Do You Sleep Less Than Seven or More Than Nine Hours per Night or Wake Up During the Night?

Healthy people need between seven and nine hours of sleep per night. Make sure you have a good-quality bed. Check to see if you have support under the center of your bed so that it doesn't sag. A good bed is firm but not rock hard.

Are You Depressed?

Feelings are a choice, but sometimes there are deeper issues that need to be addressed. Whatever you do, don't mask them with alcohol or drugs; they only get worse. Ask for help from a professional. Brain injuries can lead to depression, so this is common after car accidents. Remember to laugh daily; after all, laughter is the best medicine. Get adjusted. Adjustments remove interference and relieve stress.

Has It Been More Than a Day Since You Spent Time with God?

People cannot live on food alone; we need time with our Creator every single day. Don't just pray when times are tough; pray continually. Sin leads to sickness but repentance leads to healing.

Is There Someone You Need to Forgive?

Unforgiveness leads to poor health. It is like a slow-release poison that slowly kills us. Forgiveness, on the other hand, leads to major healing breakthroughs.

Have You Lost Your Passion for Life?

Without passion and purpose, we are just taking up space and going through the motions. Get your passion back and discover God's purpose for your life. He will use you for good things.

Do You Replenish Your Healthy Bacteria Less Than Once per Day?

We need probiotics in order to digest food and stay healthy. You probably need a supplement to get enough of these good bacteria daily. Probiotics also form part of our immune system and protect us from infections. Keep in mind that yogurt is not a great way to get probiotics.

Is Your Spine Abnormal? Is Your Nervous System Malfunctioning?

Misalignments, or subluxations, compromise the spine, which leads to disc decay and nerve damage and nerve damage leads to cell death. Get x-rays and have a chiropractor check your spine on a regular basis. Most people ignore their spine until they have pain. If a person waits until they have pain, they have waited too long. Listen to your body before it has to scream at you. Only about ten percent of our nerves are for pain, the other ninety percent are running our vital organs and tissues. Most spinal subluxations don't cause spine pain first. Usually there are other non-spinal symptoms such as fatigue, stiffness and stress.

Dr. Davis E. Lindsay

Do You Have Any Genetic Abnormalities?

You probably don't have any genetic abnormalities; they are really rare. If you do, stay positive because our thoughts can change the genetic expression of our cells.

Are You Getting Less Than Fifteen Minutes of Sunshine Daily?

You need at least fifteen minutes of sunshine daily. If you live in a northern area, you will need to supplement with vitamin D in the winter months. Or you can get a full spectrum light or use a tanning bed for 10 minutes every couple weeks.

Do You Have Any Pain That Lasts More Than Three Days?

If pain lasts for more than three days, don't ignore it; it probably is not going away on its own and will likely get worse. Pain is your brain trying to get your attention. Avoid anti-inflammatories because the first stage in healing is inflammation. It might mask the pain but you can't properly heal.

Are You Taking Any Drugs, Including Prescription Drugs (Such As Birth Control), Nonprescription Drugs (Such As Daily Aspirin), Alcohol (More Than One Drink per Day), or Illegal Drugs?

There are no safe drugs out there; every one of them is a poison. Try not to take any drugs or medications as it will only mask the problem and you will probably get worse.

Do You Have Mercury Fillings or Poor Dental Health?

Make sure you see a holistic dentist, and take care of your teeth. Poor dental health can lead to all kinds of health problems. Have a dentist safely remove the mercury from your mouth, and don't put any more in. Get a panoramic x-ray to check for rotten teeth.

The most important key to an Abundant Life

At this point I hope your head is not swimming with all the things that you might have to change. But if it is, that's good. I want you to be healthier, and sometimes getting healthier can be overwhelming.

This chapter is mostly a summary of the first thirteen chapters, with one distinction: herein lies the most important key to health. Without further ado, here is the earth-shattering truth about the way to abundant life:

> *Good health comes to those wise enough to seek it and determined enough to get it.*

All the best intentions in the world will not improve someone's health. Doing something is the key! I have found that an ounce of doing is worth more than a pound of intention. The greatest key to an Abundant Life is to be consistent.

Hopefully by now you recognize the truth in this book, but the hardest part of receiving the *abundant life* you deserve is following the *way* to get there. Knowing about good health and not making healthy choices will not result in good health. Good health is not about good luck. We are a product of our choices. We get to control our own health. The more consistent healthy choices we make, the more we give ourselves the opportunity to become healthy. Change is hard, but we do have the power to choose.

Your greatest weapon against your enslaving habits is prayer. God didn't just leave us here on our own. He is with us and will help us when we ask. He will help even when we don't ask.

Trying to change all at once is difficult and overwhelming, so most people just keep on doing what they have always done. Remember that health is a lifestyle, not some short-term goal or event. There is no time limit, but the sooner you start, the better. I wish I had known the truth sooner, but I keep on moving forward. I am healthier now than I was thirty years ago, and I am even a little healthier than last year.

Change just one thing at a time, and stick with it; that way the change becomes part of you. Exercise consistently, eat well consistently, pray consistently, get to bed at healthy time and so on.

It's also better to add healthy changes before removing unhealthy choices. For example, start eating fresh fiber first, even if you are going to eat junk food after. If you maintain those healthy choices for a year, you will be healthier in a year's time.

Think about the consequences of your choices instead of your feelings. Feelings are fleeting, but our choices stick with us. Eating junk food tastes good and feels good while we eat it but not after. Remind yourself that afterward you will not feel well. You are in control of your choices, and you can choose to be healthy.

My prayer for each person who reads this book would be that you would no longer be a slave to the lies of the world. Some of these lies are that you can't be well; that you will always need drugs or surgery to fix your problems; and that it's bad luck, bad genes, or bad germs that cause sickness.

Aging is not a disease or a cause of pain or arthritis. If we are not improving our health then we will get worse in time. This has nothing to do with our age except that it gets harder to improve as we get older. If aging did cause diseases then every person would get the same problem in the same place at the same age. That does not happen. When a person gets into their nineties or older there is definitely going to be a decline in health as the brain slowly atrophies. However, the good news even as we get older we can get better.

Our society has become enslaved in the area of health, not unlike the enslavement of the Israelites in Egypt all those years ago. The same tactics are being used: fear and propaganda. I feel that God is saying, "Let my people go." Leaving the comfort of what we know can be hard, and sometimes we will wander in the desert, but God will always be there for us. He will bring us to a better place if we follow His natural laws and decrees, because He is the God who heals.

Remember that there are three causes of all illness: deficiency, toxicity, and divine intervention. There are four stresses that relate to those three causes: spiritual stress, emotional stress, physical stress (including electromagnetic stress), and chemical stress. These stresses can come in the form of deficiencies or toxicities. The most important one is spiritual stress, the second is emotional stress, and chemical and physical stress are tied for third place.

The cure for spiritual stress is getting right with God (following His laws and commandments), fasting, praying, reading the Bible, confessing sin, and accepting Jesus Christ as your Savior.

The cure for emotional stress is acknowledging your feelings, crying, laughing, exercising, having healthy relationships, and correcting subluxations.

The cure for physical stress is exercising, avoiding injuries, maintaining good posture, sleeping, breathing properly, massage (and other types of bodywork), acupuncture and getting chiropractic adjustments.

The cure for chemical stress is eating properly, avoiding toxins in food, maintaining proper hygiene, drinking pure water, cleansing, eliminating drugs (legal and illegal), avoiding airborne toxins, not smoking, and correcting subluxations.

Remember the two most important questions to ask when faced with poor health:

1. What is the cause of these symptoms?
2. What do I need to change or do?

If your health provider won't attempt to find the cause and won't give you advice on what you need to do, fire that person and find someone who will. No one needs a doctor who just treats symptoms, you can ask Dr. Google yourself. And if you are healthier than your health care professional, go to someone else who can help you get to the next level spiritually, emotionally, and physically. After all, if the health care professional isn't healthier than you, how can he or she mentor you to better health?

These concepts are not hard to understand, but they are hard to practice consistently. You might find it helps to go back and read each chapter on its own repeatedly until you feel you have mastered that concept. Avoid television and commercials, because there are so many drug advertisements and lies designed to undermine your health and keep you enslaved. Don't live in fear of catching a disease or getting cancer. Healthy people focus on getting better, unhealthy people focus on illness. What you think about is what you will get. Don't get frustrated, hang in there, and keep trying to get a little bit better, one day at a time.

There will be times when it seems like the changes you have made are not having an effect on improving your health. If you are consistent then you will gradually see the changes. Think about the fruit trees at the beginning of spring there are no leaves on the trees, but by the end of summer not only is the tree covered in leaves but there is ripe fruit ready to be enjoyed. The same thing can happen to us when we work on ourselves.

Yours in health,
Dr. Davis Lindsay

End Notes

1   "Table 2 Percentage Using Prescription Medication, by Age Group and Number of Medications, Household Population Aged 6 to 79, Canada, 2007 to 2011," *Statistics Canada*, last modified July 17, 2015, http://www.statcan.gc.ca/pub/82-003-x/2014006/article/14032/tbl/tbl2-eng.htm 2011.

2   O. Viapiana, D. Gatti, M. Rossini, L. Idolazzi, E. Fracassi, and S. Adami, "Vitamin D and Fractures: A Systematic Review," *Reumatismo* 59 (2007): 15–19.

3   M. Terman and J. S. Terman, "Controlled Trial of Naturalistic Dawn Stimulation and Negative Air Ionization for Seasonal Affective Disorder," *American Journal of Psychiatry* 163, no. 12 (December 2006): 2126–33.

4   R. D. Levitan, "What Is the Optimal Implementation of Bright Light Therapy for Seasonal Affective Disorder (SAD)?" *Journal of Psychiatry and Neuroscience* 30, no. 1 (2005): 72.

5   K. L., Munger, S. M. Zhang, et al., "Vitamin D Intake and Incidence of Multiple Sclerosis," *Neurology* 662, no. 1 (January 13, 2004):60–65; and I. A. Van der Mei, A. L, Ponsonby, et al., "Vitamin D Levels in People with Multiple Sclerosis and Community Controls in Tasmania, Australia," *Journal of Neurology* 254, no. 5 (May 2007): 581–90.

6   M. T. Kampman, T. Wilsgaard, and S. I. Mellgren, "Outdoor Activities and Diet in Childhood and Adolescence Relate to MS Risk above the Arctic Circle," *Journal of Neurology* 254, no. 4 (April 2007): 471–77.

7   2007.

8   S. Bastuji-Garin and T. L. Diepgen, "Cutaneous Malignant Melanoma, Sun Exposure, and Sunscreen Use: Epidemiological Evidence," *British Journal of Dermatology* 146, no. s61 (April

2002): 24–30; and L. E. Beane Freeman and M. J. Van Beek, "Sunscreen Use and the Risk for Melanoma: A Quantitative Review," *Annals of Internal Medicine* 139, no. 12 (December 16, 2003): 966–78.

9   Environmental Working Group, "NIH Panel Links Vitamin A in Sunscreen to Skin Tumors" (Jan 26, 2011).

10 P. Autier, "Cutaneous Malignant Melanoma: Facts about Sun Beds and Sunscreen," *Expert Review of Anticancer Therapy* 5, no. 5 (October 2005): 821–33.

11 L. Cordain, *The Paleo Diet for Athletes* (2005).

12 N. Yoshimizu, *The Fourth Treatment for Medical Refugees: Thermotherapy in the New Century* (Honolulu: RichWay International, 2009).

13 P. Oakley, D. D. Harrison, D. E. Harrison, J. and Hass, "A Rebuttal to Chiropractic Radiologists' View of the 50 Year Old, Linear-No-Threshold Radiation Risk Model," *The Journal of the Canadian Chiropractic Association* 50, no. 3 (2006): 172–81.

14 S. Bastin and K. Henken, "Water Content of Fruits and Vegetables," *University of Kentucky* (December 1997).

15 W. S. Hodge, "Ground Water Resources of British Columbia: Ground Water Quality," Ministry of the Environment of British Columbia, May 2007, http://www.env.gov.bc.ca/wsd/plan_pro-tect_sustain/groundwater/gwbc/C03_quality.html.

16 "Calcium," *Health Canada*, October 2004.

17 L. Cordain and J. Friel, *The Paleo Diet for Athletes* (Rodale, 2005).

18 B. Pettibon, *Chiropractic and Rehabilitation Procedures Re-Invented to Correct the Spine and Posture* (Gig Harbor: Pettibon Spinal Bio-Mechnanics Institute, 2003).

19 Rubin, Paul. The Fluoride Controversy: The facts and the fiction. March 2008.

20 Paul Rubin, "The Fluoride Controversy: The Facts and the Fiction," Dr. Tom Maguire: Mercury Safe Dentists, March 2008, http://den-talwellness4u.com/layperson/fluoridefacts.html.

21 L. Dean, "Blood Groups and Red Cell Antigens," *National Center for Biotechnology Information*, 2005.

22 State Government of Victoria (Australia), *Better Health Channel*, accessed April 29, 2010, www.betterhealth.vic.gov.au.

23 James Chestnut, *Eat Well: The Innate Diet*. The Wellness Practice – Global Self Healh Corp. 2003.

24 Cordain, *The Paleo Diet for Athletes*. John Wiley and Sons 2012.

25 K. Foster-Powell, S. Holt, and J. Brand-Miller, "International Table of Glycemic Index and Glycemic Load Values," *American Journal of Clinical Nutrition 76* (2002): 5–56.

26 Canadian Diabetes Association, 2010, diabetes.ca.

27 American Diabetes Association, 2010, diabetes.org.

28 National Institutes of Health, 2013, http://ods.od.nih.gov/factsheets/Calcium-QuickFacts/.

29 *PH Brochure Rev.*, 2012, genuinehealth.com..

30 W. D. Kelley, *One Answer to Cancer* (Sterling Press, 1997).

31 N. Campbell-McBride, "Time to Get Scientific: Let's Scrap the Diet-Heart-Cholesterol Hypothesis," *CAM* (March 2007).

32 D. Melzer, et al., "Association Between Perfluoroctanoic Acid (PFOA) and Thyroid Disease in the NHANES Study," *Environmental Health Perspectives* (January 7, 2010).

33 Thyroid Foundation of Canada (April 23, 2007).

34 themastercleanse.org.

35 Arpad Pusztai, "Genetically Modified Foods: Are They a Rise to Human/Animal Health?" April 2011, actionbioscience.org.

36 International Federation for Produce Standards (IFPS), April 2011, www.plucodes.com.

37 James Chestnut, *Move Well: Innate Physical Fitness*. The Wellness Practice – Global Self Healh Corp. 2003.

38 *Nutrition Action Healthletter*, December 2009.

39 G. J. Magarian, D. A. Middaugh, and D. H. Linz, "Hyperventilation Syndrome: A Diagnosis Begging for Recognition," *West Journal of Medicine* 138 (May 1983): 733–736.

40 F. Mannello, et al., "Concentration of Aluminum in Breast Cyst Fluids Collected from Women Affected by Gross Cystic Breast Disease," *Journal of Applied Toxicology* (September 12, 2008).

41 "Mercury and Health: Fact Sheet 361," World Health Organization, accessed April 2015, http://www.who.int/mediacentre/factsheets/fs361/en/.

42 Stoner, Peter. Science Speaks – online edition. http://science-speaks.dstoner.net/index.html#c0

43 Marvin Williams, "Cast Down Sheep," *Our Daily Bread*, August 28, 2009.

44 Jeremiah, D. What are you afraid of? Tyndale House Publishers, Inc. 2013.

45 S. C. Manolagas, "Birth and Death of Bone Cells," *Endocrine Reviews* 21, no. 2 (2000): 117.

46 W. E. Winger, et al., "Possible Role of Pseudoephedrine and other Over-the-Counter Cold Medications in the Deaths of Very Young Children," Journal of Forensic Science (March 2007): 487–90.

47 B. Starfield, "Is US Health Really the Best in the World?" *JAMA* (July 26, 2000).

48 American Arthritis Foundation, January 2011, Arthritis.org.

49 P. Kjaier, et al., "An Epidemiologic Study of MRI and Low Back Pain in 13-Year-Old Children," *Spine* 30, no. 7 (2005): 798–806.

50 Y. Takatalo, et al., "Prevalence of Degenerative Imaging Findings in Lumbar Magnetic Resonance Imaging Among Young Adults," *Spine* 34, no. 16 (2009): 1716–1721.

51 N. Lender, et al., "Review Article: Associations between Helicobacter Pylor and Obesity—An Ecological Study," *Alimentary Pharmacology and Therapeutics* 40, no. 1 (July 2014).

52 S. Cullis, *The Personalized Medicine Revolution* (Greystone Books, 2015).

53 Centers for Disease Control, April 24, 2015, http://www.cdc.gov/HAI/organisms/cdiff/Cdiff_clinicians.html.

54 http://www.cdc.gov/h1n1flu/cdcresponse.htm CDC The 2009 H1N1 Pandemic: Summary Highlights, April 2009-April 2010

55 Miller, Neil Z. Vaccine Safety Manual: For concerned families and health practitioners. New Atlantean Press. Santa Fe, New Mexico. 2008 pp.60-61.

56 "WHO: Genes and Human Disease," World Health Organization, 2012.

57 Cherkas, et al., "The Association Between Physical Activity in Leisure Time and Leukocyte Telomere Length," *JAMA Internal Medicine* 168, no. 2 (2008): 154–158.